Plant-Based Diet

Plant-Based Meal Prep **+ Plant-Based** Keto Cookbook

The Complete Guide to Easy and Yummy Plant-Based Recipes, Including a 30-Day Plant-Based Meal Plan

Melissa Drew & Jorge Moore

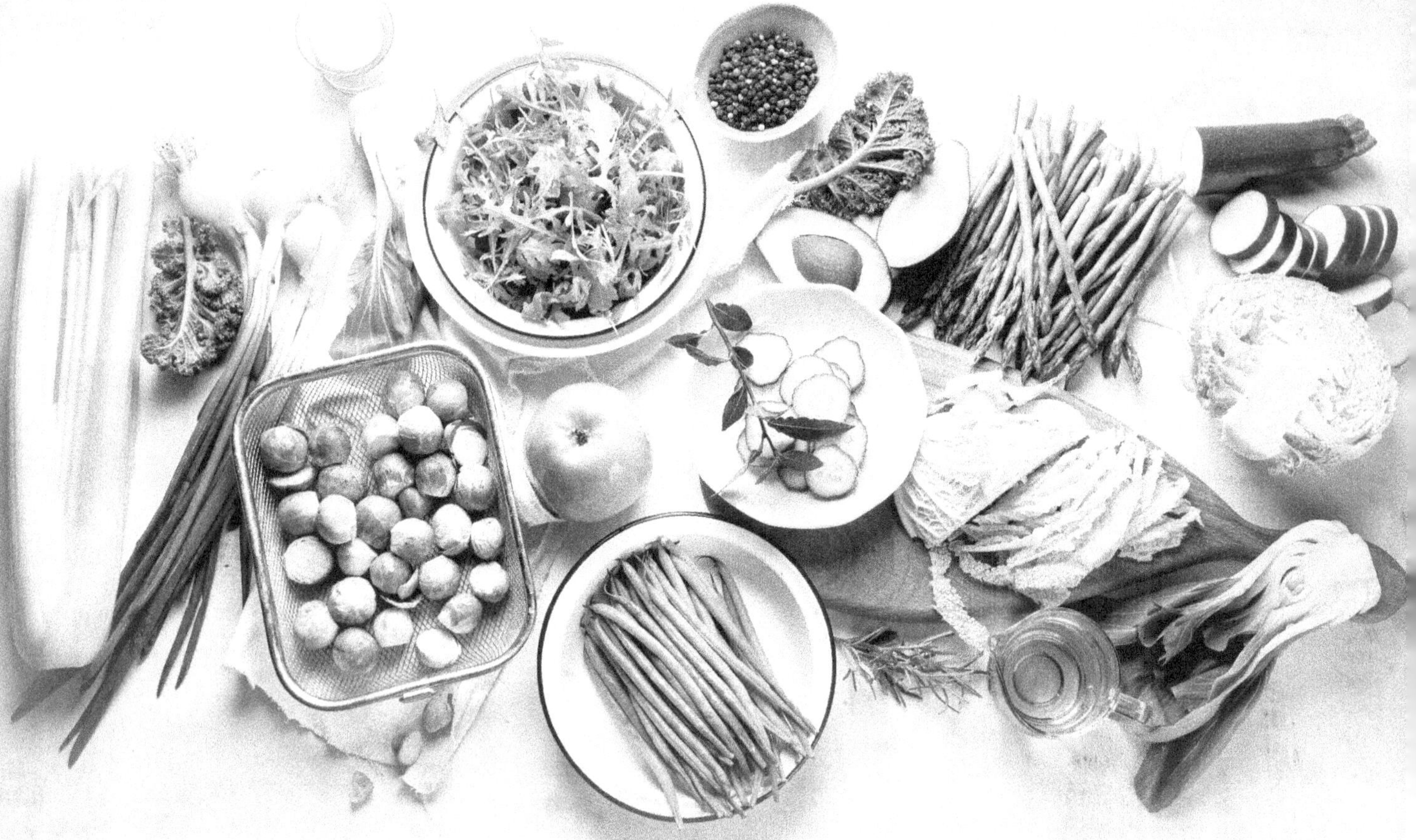

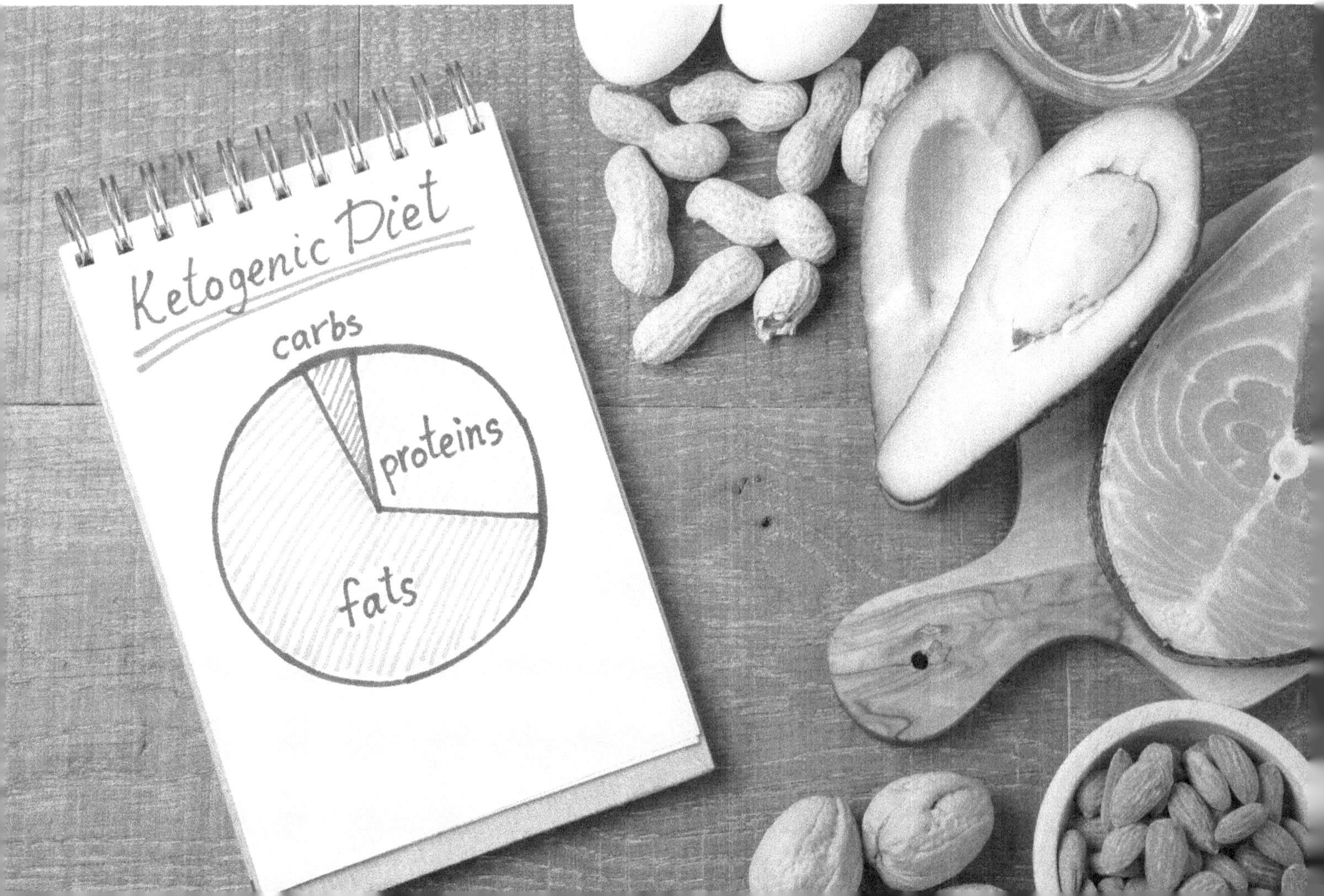

Ketogenic Diet
carbs
proteins
fats

Plant-Based Meal Prep

Easy and Delicious Recipes for Busy People. How to Approach the Plant-Based Keto. Kick-Start Healthy Eating with a 30-Day Meal Plan to Feel Satisfied and Boost Your Energy

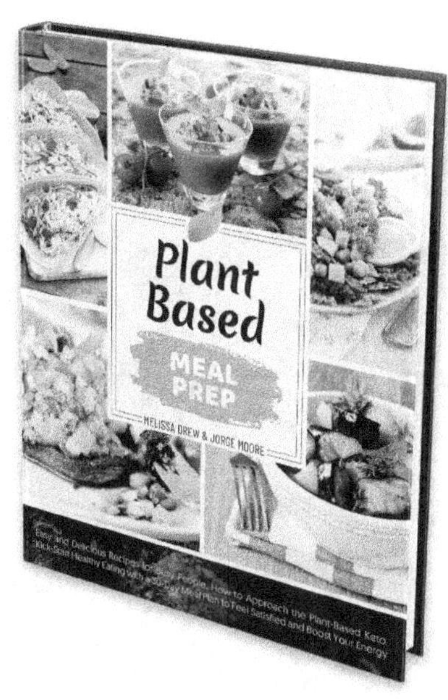

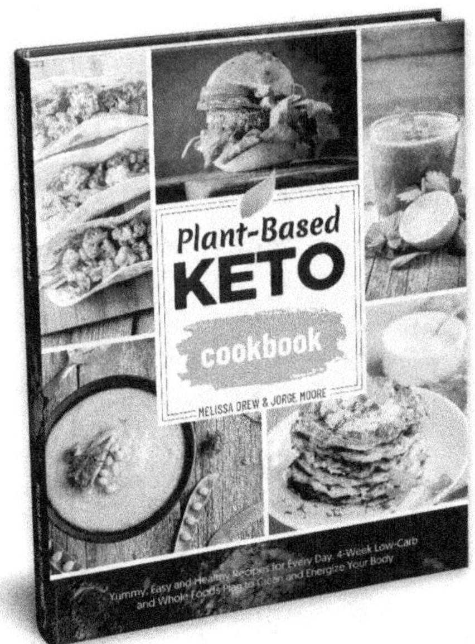

Plant-Based Keto Cookbook

Yummy, Easy and Healthy Recipes for Every Day. 4-Week Low-Carb and Whole Foods Plan to Clean and Energize Your Body

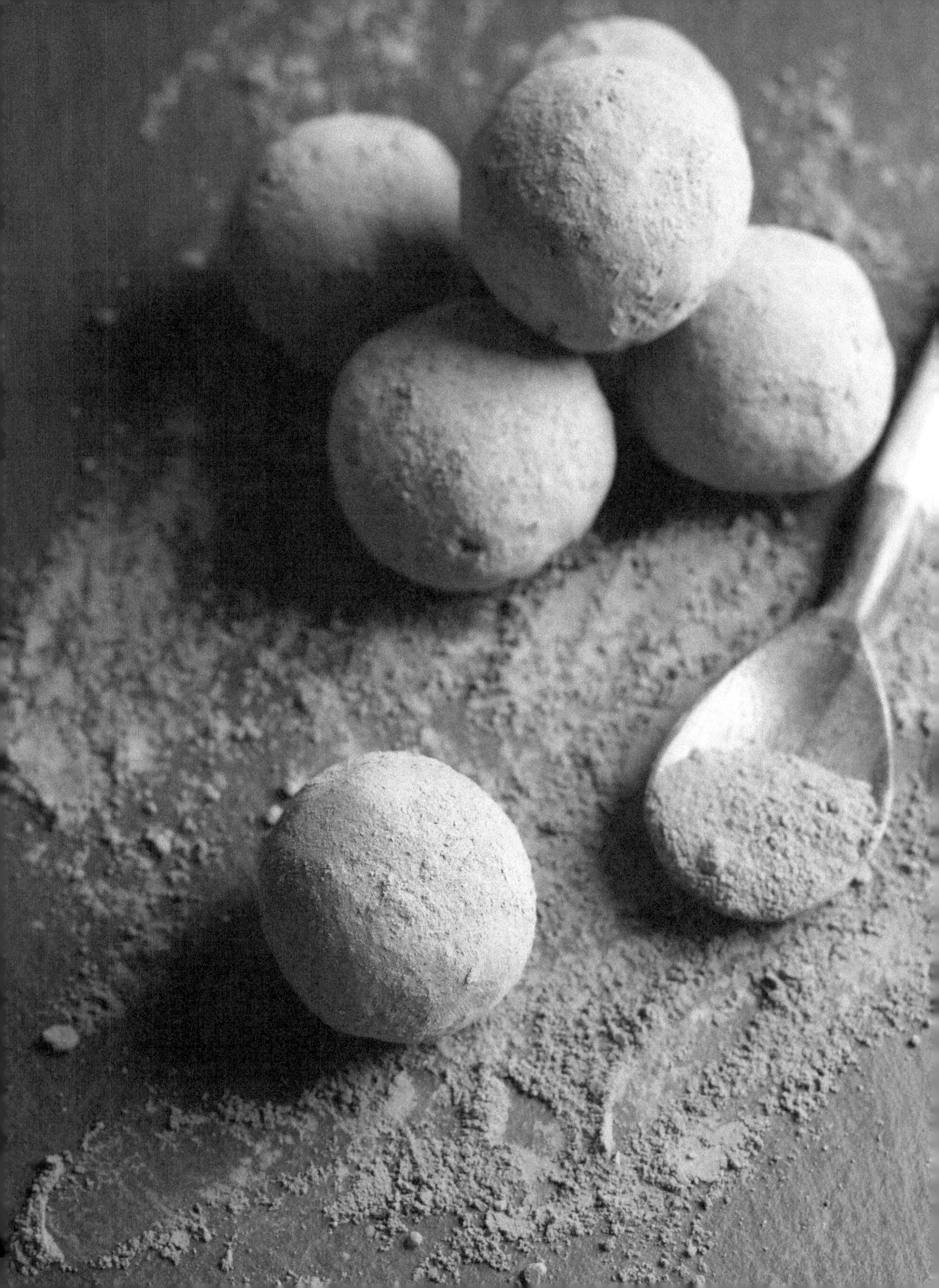

PLANT-BASED DIET

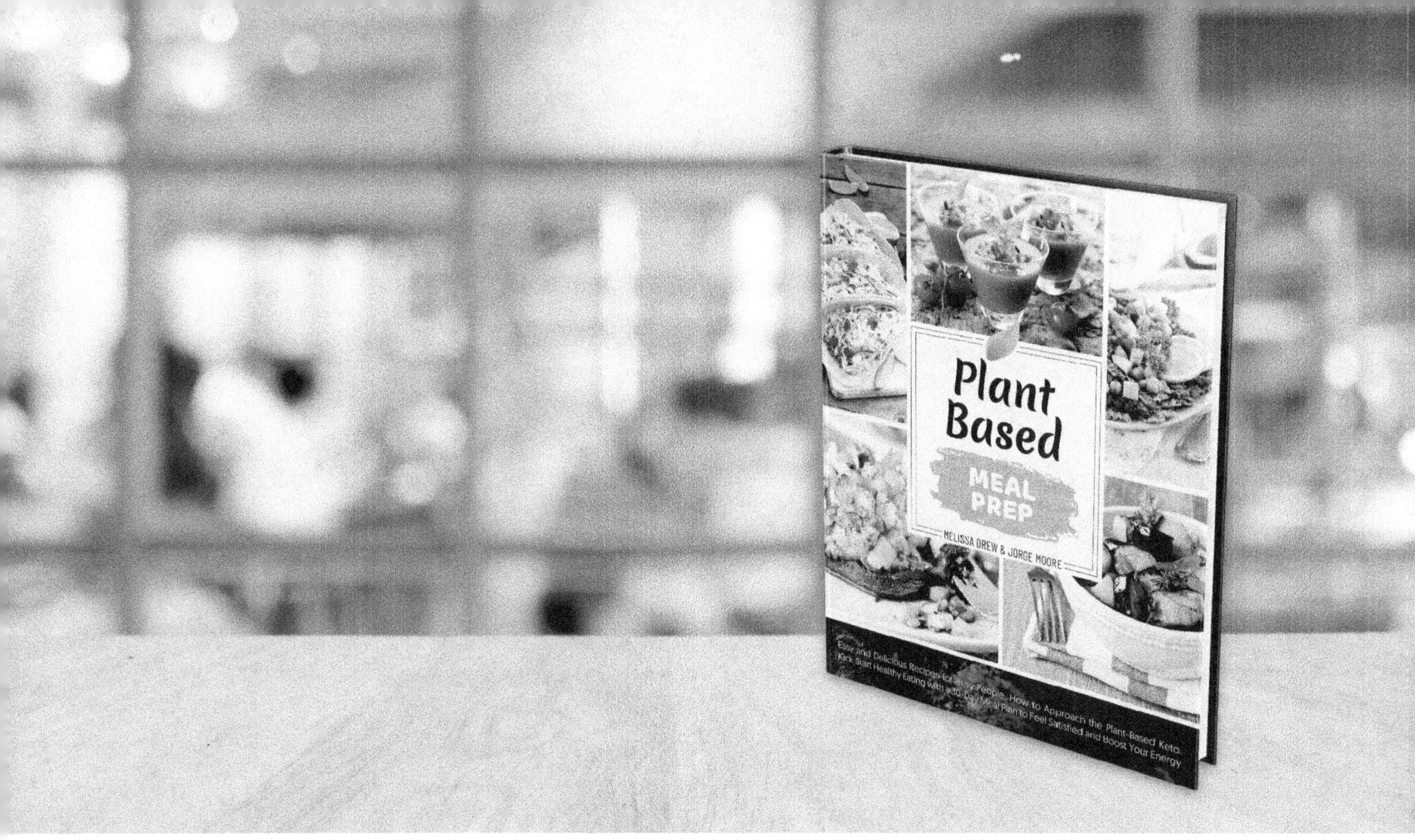

Plant-Based Meal Prep

Easy and Delicious Recipes for Busy People. How to Approach the Plant-Based Keto. Kick-Start Healthy Eating with a 30-Day Meal Plan to Feel Satisfied and Boost Your Energy

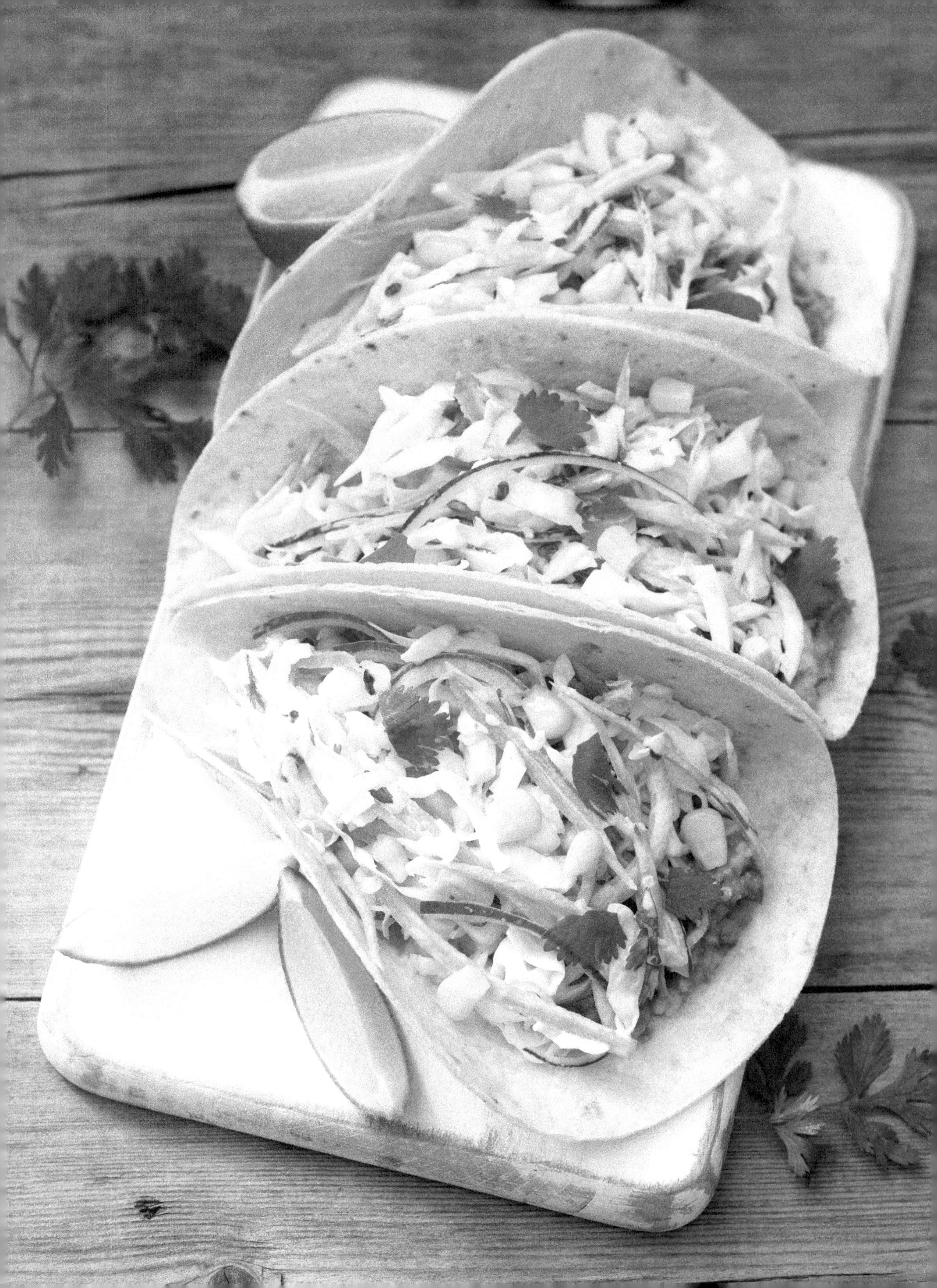

TABLE OF CONTENTS

Introduction **13**

Why You Need to Cut Back On Processed and Animal-Based Products 15

Chapter 1: Plant-Based Diet Explained **17**

Keto diet 17

Ketosis 18

Macros 19

Meal prep 20

Chapter 2: Vegan Diet and its Relation to Ketogenic Nutrition **21**

How Becoming a Vegan Can Help the Planet 24

Chapter 3: Advantages of Plant-Based Diet **29**

To the environment 30

To humans 31

Chapter 4: Shopping List for an Effective Plant-Based Diet **39**

What to avoid in a plant-based diet 40

Chapter 5: Tips on How to Resist Temptations, Control Craving and What to Do in Restaurants, or if Invited for a Dinner **41**

1) How to resist temptations 42

2) How to control cravings 44

3) What to do in restaurants 44

4) What to do when invited for dinner 45

Chapter 6: Weekly Plan **47**

Tips to incorporate into your new Plant-Based-Keto diet Plan 50

FAQS to know before you start the Plant based-Keto diet 51

Chapter 7: Breakfast Recipes **53**

Vegetable Hash 54

Flaxseed Pancakes 55

Avocado Breakfast Bowl 56

Coconut & Strawberry Bars 57

Spicy Hash Browns 58

Cantaloupe Smoothie Bowl 59

Flaxseed Porridge 60

Berry & Cauliflower Smoothie 61

Quinoa & Chocolate Bowl 62

Flaxseed & Blueberry Porridge 63

Green Mango Smoothie 64

Eggplant Hash Browns 65

Coconut & Strawberry Smoothie 66

Kiwi Slushie 67

Pumpkin Chia Smoothie 68

Breakfast Cereal 69

Walnut Porridge 70

Chia Seed Smoothie 71

Avocado & Strawberry Bowl 72

Mango Smoothie 73

Granola 74

Fruity Oatmeal 75

Chapter 8: Lunch Recipes **77**

Parsley Salad 78

Watercress & Blood Orange Salad 79

Avocado & Radish Salad 80

Zucchini & Lemon Salad 81

Lentil Potato Salad 82

Olive & Fennel Salad 83

Baked Okra & Tomato 84

Red Pepper & Broccoli Salad 85

Mediterranean Wrap 86

Cauliflower & Apple Salad 87

Mac & "Cheese" 88

Summer Chickpea Salad 89

Edamame Salad 90

Corn & Black Bean Salad 91

Butter Bean Hummus 92

Spinach & Orange Salad 93

Fruity Kale Salad 94

Chapter 9: Soups and Stews **95**

Black Eyed Peas Stew 96

Red Lentil Soup 97

Quinoa with Nectarine Slaw 98

Thai Squash Soup 99

White Bean & Spinach Soup 100

Cabbage & Beet Stew 101

Chapter 10: Dinner Recipes **103**

Sesame Bok Choy 104

Tofu & Asparagus Stir Fry 105

Tomato Gazpacho 106

Simple Chili 107

Cauliflower Rice Tabbouleh 108

Dijon Maple Burgers 109

Grilled Eggplant Steaks 110

Sushi Bowl 111

Cauliflower Steaks 112

Pesto & Tomato Quinoa 113

Ratatouille 114

Stuffed Bell Pepper 115

Black Bean Burgers 116

Fried Pineapple Rice 117

Tofu Poke 118

Conclusion **119**

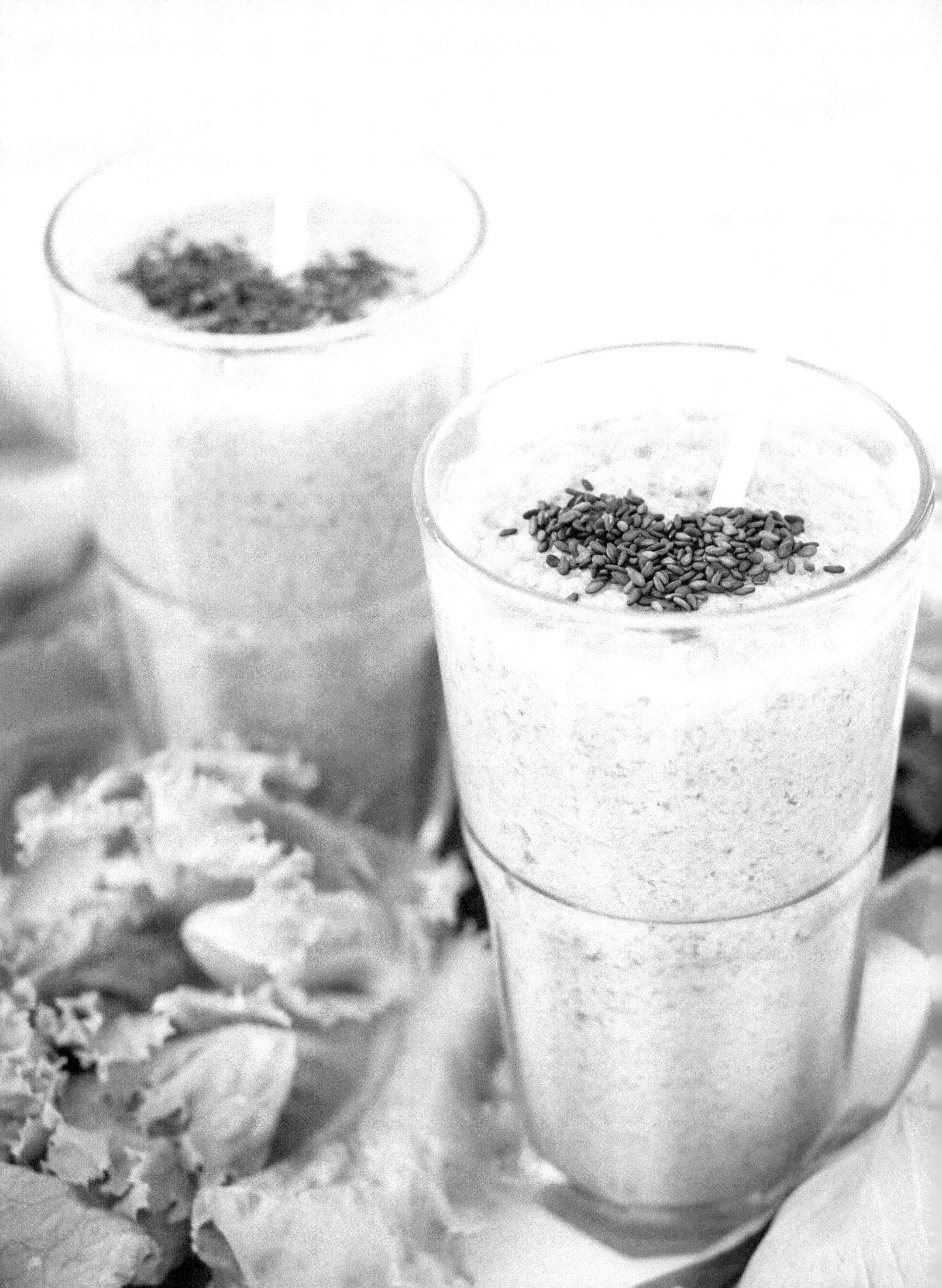

Introduction

Many people have researched and realized that the best to way to adopt a healthier lifestyle is to get into a plant-based diet. This is not an idle statement to make because experts have tried various diets before reaching the conclusion that a plant-based diet is probably the healthiest. These trials have included –

- Fasting intermittently;

- Experimenting with a low carb diet;

- The 6-meals-a-day diet;

- All protein Diet; and

- No sugar diet.

While all these diets have shown merits, a plant-based diet has trumped them all and emerged victorious in all its green and leafy glory. The major benefits of a plant-based diet include a body that is slimmer, stronger, healthier and more energetic. Not just that, because of all the healthy nutrients that the body is getting, a plant-based diet is said to improve life expectancy as well.

Of course, inherently, there are no complications to following this diet. It is simple and easy to incorporate. However, because most people have not grown up with this diet, it is the change that can seem intimidating and might make matters seem more difficult than they actually are.

There is no shame in admitting that change is daunting, and if you are planning to move to a plant-based diet, you're not the only one scared by this change. A little patience and a bit of guidance would help you embrace this diet and welcome your healthier life.

A lot of people are talking about it, but there is still a lot of confusion about what a whole food plant-based diet really means. Because we break food into its macronutrients: carbohydrates, proteins, and fats; most of us get confused about how to eat. What if we could put back together those macronutrients again so that you can free your mind of confusion and stress? Simplicity is the key here.

Whole foods are unprocessed foods that come from the earth. Now, we do eat some minimally processed foods on a whole foods plant-based diet such as whole bread, whole wheat pasta, tofu, non-dairy milk and some nuts and seed butter. All these are fine as long as they are minimally processed. So, here are the different categories:

Whole grains

Legumes (basically lentils and beans)

Fruits and vegetables

Nuts and seeds (including nut butter)

Herbs and spices

All the above-mentioned categories make up a whole foods plant-based diet. Where the fun comes in is in how you prepare them; how you season and cook them; and how you mix and match to give them great flavor and variety in your meals. There are chapters in this book dedicated to plant-based recipes which can give you an idea of what you can whip up really quick in your kitchen or those special meals you can prepare for the family.

Now, some people might say, "well, I can't eat soy" or "I don't like tofu" and so on. Well, the beauty of a whole food plant-based diet is that if you don't like a certain food, like in this case, soy, then you don't have to consume it. It is not a necessary component in a whole food plant-based diet. You can have brown rice instead of oats, quinoa instead of wheat; I'm sure you catch the drift now. It doesn't really matter. Just find something that suits you.

Just because you have made the decision to adopt a plant-based diet lifestyle, doesn't mean that is a healthy diet. Plant-based diets have their fair share of junk and other unhealthy eats; case and point, regular consumption of veggie pizzas and non-dairy ice cream. Staying healthy requires you to eat healthy foods – even within a plant-based diet setting.

Why You Need to Cut Back on Processed and Animal-Based Products

You've probably heard time and time again that processed food is bad for you. "Avoid preservatives; avoid processed foods"; however, no one ever really gives you any real or solid information on why you should avoid them and why they are dangerous. So let's break it down so that you can fully understand why you should avoid these culprits.

They have huge addictive properties

As humans, we really have a strong tendency to be addicted to certain foods, but the fact is that it's not entirely our fault.

Practically all of the unhealthy eats we indulge in, from time to time, activate our brains dopamine neurotransmitter. This makes the brain feel "good" but only for a short period of time. This also creates an addiction tendency; that is why someone will always find themselves going back for another candy bar – even though they don't really need it. You can avoid all this by removing that stimulus altogether.

They are loaded sugar and high fructose corn syrup

Processed and animal-based products are loaded with sugars and high fructose corn syrup which have close to zero nutritional value. More and more studies are now proving what a lot of people suspected all along; that genetically modified foods cause gut inflammation which in turn makes it harder for the body to absorb essential nutrients. The downside of your body failing to properly absorb essential nutrients, from muscle loss and brain fog to fat gain, cannot be stressed enough.

They are loaded with refined carbohydrates

Processed foods and animal-based products are loaded with refined carbs. Yes, it is a fact that your body needs carbs to provide energy to run body functions. However, refining carbs eliminates the essential nutrients; in the way that refining whole grains eliminates the whole grain component. What you are left with after refining is what's referred to as "empty" carbs. These can have a negative impact on your metabolism by spiking your blood sugar and insulin levels.

They are loaded with artificial ingredients

When your body is consuming artificial ingredients, it treats them as a foreign object. They essentially become an invader. Your body isn't used to recognizing things like sucralose or these artificial sweeteners. So, your body does what it does best. It triggers an immune response which lowers your resistance making you vulnerable to diseases. The focus and energy spent by your body in protecting your immune system could otherwise be diverted elsewhere.

They contain components that cause a hyper reward sense in your body

What this means is that they contain components like monosodium glutamate (MSG), components of high fructose corn syrup and certain dyes that can actually carve addictive properties. They stimulate your body to get a reward out of it. MSG, for instance, is in a lot of pre-packaged pastries. What this does is that it stimulates your taste buds to enjoy the taste. It becomes psychological just by the way your brain communicates with your taste buds.

This reward-based system makes your body want more and more of it putting you at a serious risk of caloric overconsumption.

What about animal protein? Often times the term "low quality" is thrown around to refer to plant proteins since they tend to have lower amounts of essential amino acids compared to animal protein. What most people do not realize is that more essential amino acids can be quite damaging to your health. So, let's quickly explain how.

Animal Protein Lacks Fiber

In their quest to load up on more animal protein most people end up displacing the plant protein that they already had. This is bad because unlike plant protein, animal protein often lacks in fiber, antioxidants, and phytonutrients. Fiber deficiency is quite common across different communities and societies in the world. In the USA, for instance, according to the Institute of Medicine, the average adult consumes just about 15 grams of fiber per day against the recommended 38 grams. Lack of adequate dietary fiber intake is associated with an increased risk of colon and breast cancers, as well as Crohn's disease, heart disease, and constipation.

Animal protein causes a spike in IGF-1

IGF-1 is the hormone insulin-like growth factor-1. It stimulates cell division and growth, which may sound like a good thing but it also stimulates the growth of cancer cells. Higher blood levels of IGF-1 are thus associated with increased cancer risks, malignancy, and proliferation.

Chapter 1:

Plant-Based Diet Explained

The ketogenic plant-based diet is a highly hypocaloric diet with which the amount of different nutrients to be consumed is accurately calculated so that precise proportions between them are respected. Compared to other diets, the percentage of carbohydrates is reduced to around 10%; the proteins are increased only slightly, while the fat intake can reach over 60% of the kilocalories consumed. In this way, the mobilization of the stored fats for energy production and the appearance of a particular metabolic condition called ketosis (or acetonemia), that is an accumulation in the blood of ketone bodies, substances that are formed when using fats to produce power.

This happens even when a person fasts. During fasting, in fact, the body goes through various phases to adapt to the unfavorable situation.

The sugar reserves (glycogen) present in the muscles and the liver are used; when these reserves are over we begin to use proteins, especially those of the muscles, to produce the sugar necessary for survival (through a process called gluconeogenesis); this situation stimulates the body to use fats as a source of energy with a consequent increase in ketone bodies. The ability to adapt to the unfavorable situation of fasting is a very important answer that the body puts in place in case of famine to survive; the brain, in fact, in conditions of lack of sugars, is able to use the ketone bodies to perform its important functions.

Keto diet

So you know that the Keto diet is essentially a low-carb, high-fat diet—but you'd be right to wonder just how low is "low-carb?" The traditional map for the Keto diet dictates portions in percentages based on their nutritional source. It looks something like this: eighty-five to ninety percent of your diet should come from whole, healthy fats. After that statistic, you can imagine that there isn't a lot of room for much else. Only six to ten percent of your diet is allowed to consist of protein, while the smallest portion is a tiny two to four percent carbohydrates.

In the meantime, it's incredibly helpful to know which types of foods fit in each area, and what your Keto portions should ideally look like. A typical Keto breakfast can range from steel cut oats, and berries to chocolate protein smoothies. Lunches can be huge colorful salads packed with nuts, berries, and vegetables, while dinners take on hearty spice profiles and creamy vegan sauces to make delicious warm stir-fries and vegetable macaroni. Each modern diet tends to have its own version of the classic food pyramid, but the Keto pyramid is slightly different.

When you think about what to eat on a Keto vegan diet, think about an upside-down pyramid. Your largest and biggest top section is made up of healthy fats and oils—found in nuts, seeds, avocados, and natural oils. Vegetables that aren't too starchy and vegetables that are low in carbohydrates come next, followed by nuts and berries. As a vegan on the Keto diet, you'll want to make sure that almost seventy-five percent of your fats come from plant-based fats, and that your second largest consumption is of low-starch and low-carb vegetables. Vitamins and supplements are definitely the way to go if you haven't already started taking them, but let's look a little closer at the foods you'll want to eat in order to get your nutrients naturally first.

Ketosis

As you now know, the human body has a different mechanism for breaking down and refueling that relies on fats and proteins instead of carbohydrates to keep us going. Carbohydrates like starches and fibers are packed full of sugar, and while these can be all-natural sugars, the glucose content in carbohydrate is still much higher than any other food group.

This is where the Ketogenic diet comes into play. Cellular respiration, or the process by which our cells use sugar and oxygen to create carbon dioxide and water, contains a catabolic mechanism that is perfect for breaking down fatty acids. When your body digests healthy, monounsaturated fats, each fat molecule has to be stored in a new form that is designed for later use. Fats are stored as molecules called triglycerides that are made up of one glycerol molecule and three fatty acid tails. Sugars are stored as glycogen. Both glycogen and the fatty acid tails of the stored fat molecules get processed by the Krebs cycle, one of the mechanisms of cellular respiration.

The Krebs cycle consumes acids and water in order to produce molecular bi-products that fuel the next step of energy creation with carbon dioxide as a by-product. Each molecule of stored glucose feeds two molecules of pyruvic acid into the Krebs cycle, which produces three sugar molecules each. This six carbon structure is called citric acid, and it's why the Krebs cycle is also called the Citric Acid cycle. However, something different happens when fat is broken down.

If fatty acids are fed into the Krebs cycle instead of pyruvic acid, they produce thirty-six molecules of sugar per three fatty acid chains in one triglyceride, instead of the six that one glucose molecule produces. While this is a good surplus for our bodies, it's also a surplus that we aren't designed to handle. If you've ever wondered what the "Ketone" part of the "Keto" diet is, here's the long-awaited answer. Since the Krebs cycle isn't designed to handle so many sugars all at one time, each fatty acid molecule overwhelms the system. Like a bottleneck, the Krebs cycle gets clogged with too many sugar molecules and reverts to changing each excess sugar into a three-part water-soluble Ketone body.

Macros

If you haven't already been tracking your "macros and micros" for your regular vegan diet, it's about time that you started. There is no better way to make sure you're getting the exact amount of calories, and the exact amount of nutrients, that your body needs without tracking your macros and micros.

"Macros" is an abbreviation that stands for "macronutrients," and they're what the Keto diet is based on. The three main macronutrients required for human life are carbohydrates, proteins, and fats. That's right! Tracking your macronutrients is just as easy as tracking how many grams of protein, carbohydrates, and fats you're eating in each meal. It does get a bit more complicated than that, but it's nothing you won't be able to handle.

"Micros," then, stands for "micronutrients," and these are quite different from what you might be thinking. Micronutrients are actually the vitamins and minerals that your body requires to function, and micros are often essential for macros to do their jobs. Without the help of certain minerals, our macronutrients wouldn't be able to synthesize new proteins, add in our cellular regeneration, and help move bad molecules like harmful cholesterol out of our arteries. In order to make sure you're getting your proper dosages of micronutrients, you take supplements! One of the many helpful connections between veganism and the Keto diet is that both tend to require a healthy amount of added vitamins and minerals.

Meal prep

A vegan Keto diet isn't the **most** restrictive diet out there, but it's certainly one of the more admirable challenges in the health and fitness world. Sticking to a vegan Keto diet can be hard, but meal prepping the best vegan Keto meals will make a world of difference when it comes to upholding your commitment. Many of our lives are constantly busy, and when you're trying to maintain a Keto diet, it's imperative that you eat at the same time each day—especially if you're on a fast. This might mean eating at work or packing a meal to take with you for after the gym.

Either way, preparing your necessary meals each week will give you more time to focus on your mental health and less time worrying about pounds that will melt off naturally. You'll also be able to portion out your carbs, fats, and proteins according to your Keto guidelines, which will help infinitely in organizing. As a vegan eating Keto, you'll also want to make sure that you're paying special attention to things like generated plastic waste—if you're trying to save the planet by eating less meat, it doesn't make much sense to package your snacks each day in disposable Ziploc baggies.

Glass Tupperware are the cornerstones of vegan meal prep containers, and the many different sizes and tight lids of Mason jars are perfect for taking your snacks and salads on the go. But meal preparation is more than just saving you time, money, and precious calories. Portioning out your meals is a key part of both veganism and the Keto diet because of your need to more urgently check certain nutrition boxes.

These nutrition boxes are called you macronutrients and micronutrients, and if fats, carbs, and proteins thought they were the only reason we portioned out or meals, they were very wrong. Tracking your "macros and micros" is just like making sure you don't eat too much bread in one day—except for your body, it's a lot more serious. These essential chemicals can sometimes mean the difference between a perfectly healthy body, and one that struggles to function.

Chapter 2:

Vegan Diet and its Relation to Ketogenic Nutrition

It is one thing to change your diet to lose weight, but it is a much smarter thing to commit to a lifestyle makeover like the Keto vegan diet that promotes long-term weight loss. Many of the "cleanses" and detoxes we see promoted on social media are not designed to target deeper health problems and lure dieters into a false and unhealthy sense of weight loss. Diets like this operate at a superficial level to cleanse your body of the easiest impurities you likely could have removed by just drinking water. Speaking of water, that's why these diets haven't been entirely disproven—when you crash diet, detox, or "cleanse," the weight that you **think** you're losing throughout the program is most often water weight you've simply been holding on to. Like storing sugar when we eat too much, our bodies pack on the water if we aren't hydrated enough to make our system comfortable with letting it go. This clogs our pores, skin, and internal organs with impurities that don't get flushed out because we never release the water. Detox diets and cleanses help reset your body and clean out this stagnant liquid, but you're left with no way to move forward with your weight loss. A cleanse or detox "diet" isn't a diet at all, really, since neither focuses on creating sustained patterns of healthy eating. While the Keto diet does also need to be time-regulated to make sure you don't build up too many Ketone bodies (see Chapter Two for more), a vegan Keto diet is a much more viable long-term solution than eating a regular, high carb diet with the occasional cleanse or detox. Although the Atkins diet is closest to the Keto diet in terms of guidelines and restrictions, Keto can also be compared to the modern Mediterranean diet, as well as Whole30—diets well-known for their medical benefits. Each of these regimes shares a simple and heart-healthy message: while you don't always have to refuse carbs, you should limit them, and stay away from foods high in sugar and saturated fats. Whole, monounsaturated fats help raise our levels of good cholesterol and decrease our levels of bad cholesterol. Although doctors' visits would make you believe cholesterol is only one or two numbers, cholesterol is actually a type of lipoprotein similar to the fat that has a good version, a bad version, and three other molecular arrangements. Unhealthy cholesterol comes from fats and oils that have undergone a process which makes them difficult to break down healthily. This is the cholesterol that promotes colonies of plaque that develop in your arteries and lead to atherosclerosis (the condition that occurs before a heart attack). Plaque blockages slowly cut off your circulation and force your heart muscle to work harder in order to pump the same amount of blood. This enlarging of the heart is very dangerous, and it's one of the reasons a heart-healthy diet is highly recommended by doctors. While the Keto vegan diet does have a few quirks that make it a bit more complicated, it isn't just one of the best diets for individuals who want to lose weight, keep weight off, and still eat vegan. The Keto diet is also one of the best diets for individuals who want to trust that their weight loss mechanisms are natural and sustainable. You should always make sure to check with your doctor before beginning any diet, but with the facts and guidelines in this beginner's manual, you'll be able to make an informed and knowledgeable lifestyle change for the better. Any diet based on science is bound to have merits, but with a Keto vegan diet, you're not only ensuring you won't get a dangerous dose of saturated fats—you're ensuring that any animal products treated with hormones or stimulants won't come anywhere near your body. Human beings have been eating naturally grown foods for thousands of years without added hormones and even without animal products entirely. Eliminating any possible additives as well as unhealthy carbohydrates and **too many** carbohydrates essentially eliminates the large majority of common nutritional issues. The science is there, but with the Keto vegan diet, there's more proof in the actual experience. Keep this in mind as we head into our next section, to take a look at some tips and tricks that you can use to make sure you're eating the best possible vegan diet before implicating a Ketogenic plan.

Quick Tips to Get Your Veganism in Shape for Keto

The five best supplements to take as a vegan are Calcium, Iron, Vitamin B12, Omega-3 fatty acids, and Zinc. Iron and vitamin B12 are both well-known deficiencies in just about everyone, so you can't go wrong taking them as a vegan (especially when you know that you aren't getting iron from red meat). A word of caution: when it comes to your iron, you don't have to take it for long. Our body builds up iron stores and can sustain them for an extended period, so you'll only take an iron supplement for about a month or so at a time with breaks in between. Iron is definitely one you can take yourself, but asking your general practitioner never hurts. While calcium is absolutely a mineral you can find in plants, it's a tricky one. You would have to eat a TON of kale just to make up for a few glasses of whole milk. However, calcium takes care of more than a few things in your body, which makes it necessary. Calcium strengthens your teeth and bones, helps your blood properly clot, and if you're big into getting those gains, listen up—our muscles physically cannot contract without it. Calcium is necessary for all muscle contractions throughout our bodies, and if you're planning on building strong bones **and** strong muscles, it's time for a trip to the vitamin store. Not to worry though - a supplement does just fine, and you won't have to take it forever. Make sure to take your calcium in doses smaller than 1,000 milligrams, with food, and during a different time of day than when you take your other vitamins (calcium can inhibit your body from absorbing other minerals). If you have a history of heart problems or are on medication for a heart-related condition, you should speak with your first doctor about supplementing your calcium. Although omega-3 fatty acids are found in fish, if you don't want to take fish oil, there are a few good food options instead - all you have to do is read your labels for something called "alpha-Linolenic acid." This type of non-animal derivative Omega-3 is found in all your favorite seeds like hemp, chia, and flax, et cetera. Even algae, seaweeds, and soy products contain healthy omega-3 fatty acids. But you can also find manufactured supplements from companies whose products are cruelty-free and 100% fish oil free, so you know you'll be getting a proper vegan dosage. But be sure to check your labels—not all "vegan" products are actually vegan. While it's always a great idea to look for a multi-vitamin that contains each one of these ingredients in any general amount, you shouldn't rely on your multi-vitamin alone on a vegan diet. You simply need more. Now that your body has the tools you need to burn fat, synthesize protein, and fight off infection, let's talk about balancing your vegan nutrition from a tastier perspective.

A Balanced Vegan Diet Is the Keto Key

It's also important to make sure that your vegan diet is a nice balance between healthy fats, proteins, and carbohydrates. Many vegans struggle to work out the right proportions when they first begin eating vegan, but you should always stick to limiting your carbs with each meal to no more than one-quarter cup, combined with a one-cup portion of vegetables and a 1/2 cup portion of protein. The Keto diet aims to cut almost all your carbs and starchy vegetables, so if you're the type of vegan who relies on pasta and bready foods to get you through your diet, it might be time for a change. If you're knowledgeable about your nutrition, you might be wondering about fruit; it's packed with a ton of sugar carbohydrates, so if so many other starchy vegetables are limited, is fruit? The Keto diet does actually limit ALL fruit, which might sound a little crazy and a lot hard to follow. Adjusting to eating almost no fruit (you're allowed some wiggle room, but your fruit will count towards your daily fifty grams or less) is incredibly difficult, but don't give up just yet! Fruits that are higher in carbohydrates tend to be yellow, orange, or pink, and are overall larger in size—but this isn't always the case. The easiest way to remember which fruits NOT to eat is to remember which fruits you CAN eat. Small berries are lower in carbs, and a few handfuls won't break your diet while they satisfy your sweet tooth. You'll also want to keep an eye on the amount of sugar you eat in other foods (or drink!) because the Keto diet cuts out that too. Trimming down your carbohydrate and sugar portions a few weeks before you begin the Keto diet will also help with the carb "flu" or "Keto flu" that some dieters experience when they first enter carbohydrate and glucose withdrawal. Before we jump into Keto, however, let's brush up on the best habits you should already be practicing as a healthy vegan.

How Becoming a Vegan Can Help the Planet

I am sure you've heard from many people that our planet is not in the best shape. Many people are becoming more ecologically conscious out of deep respect for our planet and the desire to make it better. Because of the wish to change things, people have begun to adopt the veganism lifestyle. While not as many people have adopted the veganism lifestyle as much as the plant based one, veganism is well on the rise and its very likely that you've either heard of it, seen a viral video online as there are hundreds of channels devoted to helping people understand the lifestyle, or even possibly seen a protest at one point as there have been quite a few at concerts or places where they believe animals are being abused.

There are so many studies done about why being a vegan can help the planet and one says that one pound of beef requires fifteen times more water to produce than a pound of soy and thirteen percent more fossil fuel. It's a sobering thought to think of our resources that way. By stopping your use of animal products, you can begin to help with these issues.

Being a vegan will also spare hundreds or even thousands of animals in your lifetime.

Our human population keeps getting bigger and it is expected that it will grow by three billion. It is also said that there will be plans to help poorer countries get more meat to feed their people which means in the next few decades, we will need more animals to eat. Many people believe that this is going to be a massive food crisis later on. Also, it has been said that because plant based survive mostly on vegetables and not meat, they need less living space. This means that they could survive on less land than those who survive mostly on meat. A good example of this would be a family that lives in Bangladesh which is living off of just rice, vegetables, and other plant-based items. They would need less land and farming because they wouldn't be raising cattle, pigs, or the other animals that carnivores and omnivores consume daily. However, the average family that lives in America can consume around two hundred and seventy pounds of meat in just a year, so they would need twenty times as much land.

It is said that about thirty percent of the available surface of the planet that is ice-free, is being used by livestock. Unfortunately, there are one billion people who can't eat and go hungry every day and livestock consume most of the world's crops. Another downside is that our hunger for meat has led to desertification and soil erosion and it puts so much extra stress on people's homelands. Overgrazing from the uplands of Ethiopia to the mountains of Nepal or the down lands of southern England also causes flooding and great losses of fertility.

It is said that the figures that have been studied need to be treated with caution. Animal manure can actually revitalize the soul and there are millions of animals that live on marginal land which is quite unsuitable for crops.

Another thing to think about is that in some farms where they raise cattle for meat, they are ensured to be raised in a way that packs the most meat on them as they possibly can before they are killed for us. This is not true in countries that are not as well off. Cattle in poorer countries is essential for some people's way of life. It ensures they have a job and food. Without it, they wouldn't.

There is also so much water used to raise animals. Studies have shown it takes about nine thousand liters of water or in pounds, that's twenty thousand, to produce one pound of beef. Additionally, to produce one liter of milk, nearly one thousand liters of water are needed. A broiler chicken takes much less than beef, but it still needs one thousand five hundred liters of water. Another example of how much water is used is pigs. Pigs are said to be some of the thirstiest animals. If you're looking at it, an average sized pig farm in North America will have about eighty thousand pigs. Those eighty thousand pigs need nearly seventy-five million gallons of much-needed water over the course of a single year. That number grows exponentially when you think of the size of the farms in bigger cities. If you think about that for a second, that is a lot of water, and that could be used for other things. As a plant based, you will have the knowledge that you're not contributing to those numbers. You will be saving so much water simply by not eating any of the meat that uses so much of our water.

There has been the saying that water is not an infinite resource and the earth does not have enough for ages. The information varies from source to source but the guesswork of how much water it takes to produce just one kilo of beef can vary from thirteen thousand liters to even one hundred thousand liters. Clearly, that's a massive amount of water being used for just one kilo. Imagine how much water is being used for a city's supply of meat or an entire continent. To take your perception even further, it only takes one thousand to two thousand liters to produce one kilo of wheat. That's a far cry from the thirteen thousand it takes for beef, isn't it?

We've all heard of global warming, right? The vice president has mentioned it, celebrities have mentioned it, and it's everywhere you look. Many children learn in school about the damage to the ozone layer and celebrate Earth Day and try to be clean and help the planet. Many people have theorized that animals produce more greenhouse gases than all of the cars on the planet. That's a lot of gas. They further theorize that by adopting a plant-based diet and not eating the animals, you can vastly reduce the number of greenhouse gases and save the planet from getting hurt more than it already is. While people are discovering if we can reverse the damage, it has been told to us that we can try and stop the planet from getting worse. So if they say adopting a vegan diet is going to help the issue of greenhouse gases, imagine how much more you'd be helping as a vegan!

Along with greenhouse gases, sheep and cows make up about thirty-seven percent of the methane that is being emitted into our air. These statistics for methane are twenty-three times as warming as the CO2 that's being emitted. Thirty-seven percent is nearly half of the methane emissions. That's a completely insane amount of emissions. We need to reduce this number as much as possible and quickly. Acid rain is being contributed to as well by ammonia emissions which thanks to the livestock industry is said to be sixty-four percent. Manure from the animals was consuming produces sixty-five percent of nitrous oxide that's human-related or caused. This is about three hundred times the global warming potential of CO2 that's produced. A vegan diet can cut these numbers down as well and begin to reduce emissions simply from taking the meat out of your diet.

Richer countries that are water stressed such as South Africa, and Libya or Saudi Arabia say that it makes sense that poorer countries grow food to conserve their water resources. Some countries are even trying to help others by growing their cows in their countries then sending them to others.

We could be poisoning the earth. When animals excrete manure and you have hundreds or thousands in a tiny area, the manure is funneled along with the urine into a waste lagoon that can hold massive amounts. Some hold as much as forty million gallons. The cesspools often break and leak or overflow because they are holding so much, and this pollutes water supplies and underground water supplies as well. It also pollutes rivers with phosphorus and nitrates along with nitrogen. There are thousands of miles of rivers in Europe, Asia, and the United States that are polluted each and every year.

The sheer number of animals that people need or choose to eat is harming the earth in other ways as well. We could be hurting our planet's biodiversity. The definition of biodiversity tells us that it is the variety of life in a particular habitat or in the world or a particular ecosystem. The reason that biodiversity is important is that it boosts productivity in an ecosystem where all species, no matter how big or small, all have a part to play. An example to help you understand would be if you imagine a large number of plant life or species. Larger plant life equals a larger variety of crops. If we have greater species diversity, we are ensuring sustainability for all life forms. But not just sustainability; natural sustainability too.

We are spoiling the oceans of the world and killing innocent sea life. When so much excess waste gets dumped into the water, the fish begin to die for no reason other than humans are polluting the only home they have.

There are nearly four hundred dead zones and they range in all different sizes. They've ranged from one square kilometer to over seventy thousand square kilometers. They've been identified from the South China Sea to the Scandinavian fjords. The culprit of these dead zones is not only animal farming, but it is one of the worst as it causes so much damage.

Animal waste is making us more prone to getting sick because many of the pathogens in animal waste include E. coli bacteria that can be transferred so easily; hundreds could get infected and cryptosporidium. Cryptosporidium is a genus of apicomplexan parasitic alveolate. It can cause gastrointestinal illness or respiratory illness. The main problem this causes is watery diarrhea and it comes with or without a cough. If you do get this cough, it will be pretty persistent. In addition, another problem with livestock is that they don't grow fast enough or have enough meat for the farmers and each year, they need more and more meat. So they have to resort to new methods. Those methods for getting them to produce more also have an effect on us and how we get sick.

Another bad thing about eating meat? The quantity of meat that people consume is absolutely staggering. Studies over time have shown that on average, a British carnivore will eat about or even over eleven thousand animals in their lifetime. These animals include twenty-eight ducks, one thousand one hundred and fifty-eight chickens, three thousand five hundred ninety-three shellfish, four cattle, six thousand one hundred and eighty-two fish, eighteen pigs, thirty-nine turkeys, one rabbit, twenty-three lambs and sheep, and one goose.

The plant based and vegans are speaking up about this saying that because of this, the meat eaters have increased chances of becoming obese. They also say that heart disease and cancer can come from this as well.

There are so many problems with this world because the meat-eaters were consuming many of them listed above. In your life as a vegan, you can save hundreds of animals from the fate of being hurt and you can begin to help the planet from these horrible issues that have been arising from livestock. A vegan benefits everyone because you're not contributing to the production of these animal farms and they take it a step further by removing any animal item from their life which means they benefit the planet even more.

Chapter 3:

Advantages of Plant-Based Diet

One of the main reasons people become vegans is to help the animals as they feel its morally and ethically wrong to eat them because it's cruel and inhumane. They also have moral and ethical issues about how eating animals effects the planet. But believe it or not, while there are many benefits to being vegan and adopting a vegan ketogenic diet, there are also downsides not just for your health but for the planet as well.

The planet has many poor countries. Some so poor that they feed their children dirt before they go to school because it's all their community has. Some so poor that they are dying without proper water. In some of these poor countries, they need all the meat they can get because they may not be able to nourish their people with anything else. The same situation is present in countries where grazing is efficient because they don't have any land that is suitable for growing or sustaining crops.

Another reason it might not be the best is that if we all stop eating meat, the planet would be overpopulated with animals and then the emissions would grow higher because their still producing manure but now, there's more of it and the wheat that could be feeding starving people is being used to feed animals instead. This sounds heartless and like the animals should be eaten for meat, which is not what I am saying at all. The animals deserve to live as any other creature. We are merely presenting facts.

Remember the countries that don't have soil that can produce good crops? As people will be eating less meat, that means they will need to eat more plants. In those lands that have soil which won't produce, the sheep, cattle, and goats are actually helping make that inedible grass and turning it into edible milk and meat for the people. In some countries, that milk and meat is their only source of protein and fat to keep them nourished. If you take it away, what do they have left if they don't have crops?

Also, the land mostly used for nuts, fruits, and vegetables is cultivated cropland. Grazing cropland is usually unsuitable for attempting to grow crops but is actually really good at feeding animals that we use for food such as cattle. The last type of cropland that we have is called perennial cropland. This is good for grain, hay, and other types of crops that are alive year-round. What they do is harvest these crops multiple times before dying. The reason the vegan diet sticks out here is that it's the only diet that doesn't use all of the lands. It specifically doesn't use perennial cropland which would waste the chance to produce more food for the people of the planet.

The livestock industry, though hated by some, also creates a livelihood or jobs and means of support for over one billion of the world's poor families and employs over one point three billion people. Without the livestock industry, those families would be out of a job.

The shocking thing about greenhouse gasses is that while most people believe that meat is causing many greenhouse emissions (and they are, believe it or not), it has been proven that some vegetables can cause just as many gasses as meat! Studies have shown that if you're going by calories, making lettuce can create as much greenhouse emissions as beef. It has been shown that lettuce generates about three times what pork or fresh fish does in greenhouse gasses. That's crazy, right?

To the environment

Food waste is also a really big problem that takes a toll on the environment. Fruits and vegetables tend to be one of the highest wasted foods at forty percent to the only thirty-three percent that meat does. That's only a seven percent difference but it does add up. One issue that makes these findings difficult is that it also varies from country to country with what people throw away and waste. Some things are agreed upon though and it's what makes the science easier to comprehend. Perishability is also another argument. Fruits, vegetables, and a lot of other things that vegans need to survive perish very quickly and most people are more likely to throw away these food items than dairy or meat because they've gone bad. So while a vegan world would benefit in many ways, it would also hurt in a few ways as well especially if it's not sustainable for many people because of where or how they live.

To humans

There are also health problems that can arise from you being a vegan and a ketogenic. We will start with the problems that arise from being a vegan first.

Osteoporosis is a serious health issue that can arise if you're not eating properly. Calcium is a very important nutrient that you shouldn't ignore and yet, unfortunately, there are many in the vegan lifestyle that can do just that. This can cause your bones to become weak and result in fractures and damage you might not be able to repair at all. Ways to keep your calcium up as a plant based are to eat items like kale and Chinese cabbage or spinach and broccoli. High potassium items with high magnesium can reduce blood acidity. You can find items like this in the fruits and vegetables you would just need to check. Lowering the blood acidity is helpful because you are lowering the chances of excreting calcium through your urine.

Regardless of what you eat on this particular diet, you might still need a supplement if you're not getting the things you need for your body. For example, studies have shown that most vegans do not get enough vitamin D and may need to take a supplement to correct that. Since this includes dairy products, vegans don't have the option of not taking one as plant-based do, and they have no choice but to take a supplement to make sure they are getting the right amount in their body or it can be detrimental to their health.

One of the biggest debates about the ketogenic diet is whether going into ketosis is safe. Ketosis can actually be dangerous when your ketones build up. It can lead to high levels of dehydration and it is said that it can change the chemical balance of your blood. Another problem is if ketosis goes too far, the body can go into ketoacidosis. This is what happens when ketones build up in your blood. When they build up in your blood, it becomes acidic. This can cause your body to go into ketoacidosis which can cause you to fall into a coma or die. People with diabetes are especially susceptible to ketoacidosis if they don't take enough insulin or if they're injured or sick. People can also fall into ketoacidosis when they have an overactive ethmoid or be caused by starvation.

It's very important to understand that if your feeling tired or have flushed skin, throwing up, confusion, pain in your stomach, fruity smelling breath, feeling thirsty or even urinating a lot, these are all signs of ketoacidosis and you should call a doctor right away. Especially when you have diabetes, the symptoms may start slowly with throwing up, but the process speeds up quickly in just a few hours. So, when you're in ketosis, you need to make sure you don't fall into ketoacidosis because it can lead to fatal sickness.

Lastly, another reason to be cautious is that in a ketogenic diet, your insulin levels begin to go down. This causes your body to shed water and sodium. When the body does it, this is beginning to do what is called reduced bloat. It can also cause dehydration and lightheadedness or constipation and headaches. Low sodium is bad for the body because if your sodium and electrolyte levels are low, you can have muscle weakness and changes in blood pressure. More scarily, your heartbeat can become irregular.

Dehydration is also a big issue with the ketogenic diet because, in the first two weeks, you're losing water and electrolytes. It's also known as a water flushing diet because there is a lessening of inflammation. There is also a reduction of glycogen stores in your liver and muscles. To keep yourself from getting dehydrated, you might need to drink about two liters or more a day. You should start when you begin cutting the carbs in your diet because of being ketogenic.

Social media is also dangerous on this diet or honestly any diet. Many people think they're helping or being supportive. Those people are alright as long as they're giving the proper advice. Others like tearing others down and giving bad advice. One big problem that many people encounter unfortunately is bad advice. If you go on social media, there are so many people trying to tell you how to live your life and how you should go about it. Now, to be fair, most of these people think that they are helping. Some of them are and they've done their research to make sure that they are giving good advice and they've talked to doctors to make sure that the information they are giving people is good information. Others, however, can be causing damage to people and making them sick. For example, one social media user says she only eats a certain number of calories a day. If you do your homework, you'll realize those are eating disorder levels and not healthy. As many young women and men watch her channel, this person could be potentially harming thousands of young people and they could think that eating disorders are alright when they are not. Eating disorders affect so many people these days. When you're dieting, it's so important to make sure you're taking in the proper calories so that you don't fall into dangerous territories. You will also need to eat a variety of foods. This prevents you from falling into other dangerous territories like orthorexia.

Others on social media say that you can eat over five thousand calories a day (most of which are certain types of sugar), not work out, and you will lose weight and not have health problems. That is simply untrue and that can be potentially life-threatening advice. Some people have diabetes and that much sugar can put them into ketoacidosis which can be fatal. The scary part about this is that for diabetics, it can become fatal in a matter of hours. That's a terrifying thought. Even normal people who don't have any issues can be severely damaged by this advice. You can gain weight which causes many health problems on its own; you cannot ingest that many calories and not work out and expect that you won't put on any pounds at all. You will because you're consuming so many calories a day. There are many other problems with this advice as well and people shouldn't follow extreme diets because it's not safe and it's misleading to give people advice without making sure that it's safe for the people who are listening to you.

Everyone can get on social media these days. We live in a digital world and children and teenagers younger and younger are taking advice from the net and not their parents. This is not a good thing. There is so much information on the internet that isn't true and even more dangerous to impressionable young minds. People on the net or social media say that they can say what they want and shouldn't have to worry about what they say but they should. They are considered role models to people around the world and with a society so crazed about diets, we need to understand what's real information that is the right information and what is false and dangerous to our health.

Fast food options for vegans are not the healthiest either and they're kind of difficult to come by sometimes. So, when going out into this diet, you'll need to be careful about where you go. If you live in certain areas where veganism is more prominent, then you'll probably have more access to vegan-friendly restraints. Whereas if you live somewhere where it's more meat inclined, not so much. In these cases, your supermarkets will probably also have a harder time having good vegan options as well which can be a pain.

If you do manage to find a vegan option at a fast food restraint, you still need to remember your golden rule. Check the ingredients and know the calorie information as well as your micros and macros. Just because it is a vegan option doesn't mean that its ketogenic as well. You need to make sure that whatever you're going, go for the healthy option. Remember there are foods on this diet that you can eat but they're not healthy for your goals.

Most ketogenic also make what is called a fat bomb. This is a very popular trend in the Keto world, but it may not be the safest one. The 'fat bombs' are usually high in fat, of course, with a moderate amount of either artificial or natural sweetness. Keto dieters usually refer to fat bombs as a treat, snack, or Soups and stew. Some use it before a workout. Some use it as a fat dense snack or a way to curb their sweet tooth. With the Keto diet, you're trying to cut sugar and carbs. You're trying to eat cleaner. These fat bombs are usually ninety percent fat or even more. The fat from these bombs commonly comes from coconut milk or from dairy. While most use it as a snack or Soups and stew, some actually use it for a meal replacement. There is so much fat in these bombs that the calories for a single one can be anywhere from two hundred and fifty calories to five hundred calories. We know that Keto dieters strive for higher fat but depending on your calorie intake for the day, you're using a big chunk of your calories for a small little goodie.

The goal of the Keto diet is to achieve ketosis. When you reach for snacks like you would with a fat bomb, it could mean you're not in a state of ketosis any longer. Meaning, fat bombs are basically promoting snacking unnecessarily. Boiled eggs are a better way to respond to hunger. Your body needs to take its own time on this diet and there is no quick fix. If you suddenly begin to consume large amounts of fat, that's not going to make you adjust quicker.

The Keto diet's success is the result of hormones; one hormone in specific as a matter of fact. It's called leptin. Leptin reacting to a lack of blood sugar in your body results in your body using stored fat for energy. The fat that is consumed for the energy would be used before the stored fat. This means that the benefits of fat bombs are diminished in terms of fat loss. This is because while you could be maintaining ketosis, you're fueling your ketones with the wrong thing. You're fueling them with fat bombs instead of an extra arm, stomach, or thigh fat.

Insulin and leptin are opposing hormones in your body. One tells the body to stop storing fat, the other tells the body to store fat. Many people are concerned with insulin and insulin resistance. But a higher priority needs to be given to leptin. In the human body, any hormone that you overproduce decreases the bodies sensitivity to it. So in a body that has excess fat, the hormone leptin is being overused. The impact of leptin resistance in the body is that the body does not know how or when to stop storing fat. So the fat could come from frying oil or coconut oil, but it wouldn't matter.

The people that are encouraging fat bombs and swearing by them fail to realize or recognize that leptin resistance in the body (though improved) when you're in ketosis, is still a really serious hormonal adaptation. This adaptation isn't going to be reversed by consuming high amounts of fat.

Another thing nutritionist say is that if you want to slim down, a ketogenic diet is not the best way to do this. It's considered extreme and nutritionists warn it may not be healthy. Others say that it's not sustainable for people and they believe it's just not a good diet for you. Since this diet is also low in fiber, it's been said that that can cause digestive issues with your body. They believe if you do a more balanced diet, it will be better for your future diets and goals.

Many talk about it, but few know it. The ketogenic plant based diet is mainly based on the mechanism of ketosis (a symptom of an altered fatty acid metabolism) and involves the reduction or elimination of carbohydrates from the diet for a short period. By reducing or eliminating them drastically, and increasing proteins and lipids, fat accumulation can be reduced to use it for energy purposes: the decrease in glucose levels will ensure that the body will be forced to draw energy directly from fat.

The Health Benefits of the Ketogenic Plant based Diet

The benefits of a ketogenic diet are similar to those that can be obtained from any poor, or even lacking, carbohydrate diet. However, in this case, the results could be greater, considering that ketogenic diet results in a significant drop in protein. The benefits that can be obtained by following the ketogenic diet can be found not only in weight loss, which is accelerated but also in the reduction of acne (among the causes, excess sugar that could cause hormonal imbalance).

And again, this type of diet - which focuses entirely on the significant reduction of carbohydrate intake - could represent, for people with cancer, an adequate complementary treatment to chemotherapy, without forgetting its possible support in the prevention and treatment of diseases important as Parkinson's and Alzheimer's, but also a valid ally for those who suffer severely from sleep disorders.

Following a diet low in carbohydrates and rich in lipids helps to lose weight, but above all, according to a growing number of studies, it helps to reduce the risk factors related to diabetes, cardiovascular diseases, and epilepsy, to name a few diseases. The ketogenic plant-based diet encourages the consumption of fresh and natural foods, such as meat, fish, vegetables and fats and healthy oils, and at the same time provides a strong limitation of processed and preservative-rich foods. It is a sustainable and pleasant diet, even in the long term. After all, how does he not like a diet that includes eggs and bacon for breakfast?

Frequent studies show that the ketogenic plant-based diet, compared to other food programs, helps to lose more weight, to increase energy levels, and to feel a sense of satiety that lasts longer. The last two aspects are due to the fact that most of the calories come from lipids, very caloric substances, and slow digestion. Consequently, those who eat ketogenic normally consume fewer calories because they feel full longer and therefore need to eat less and less frequently.

How Does the Ketogenic Plant base Diet Lead to Weight Loss?

Usually, the body gets its energy from the carbohydrates consumed during the day and which are necessary for the proper functioning of the body. In the ketogenic diet, carbohydrates are extremely limited, and the body begins to tap into its stores of carbohydrates stored in the muscles and liver called reserves of glycogen. As each gram of glycogen is bound to 3-4 g of water in the body, the significant weight loss at the beginning of the ketogenic plant-based diet is largely a loss of water. When glycogen stores are depleted, the body naturally begins to use lipids or fats to produce energy. Off, when the body uses lipids in the absence of carbohydrates, it produces waste called ketone bodies.

Why Switch to A Ketogenic Plant based Diet Style?

When you follow a ketogenic plant-based diet, the body becomes efficient at burning fat for energy. This is advantageous for many reasons, not least the fact that fats have more than double the calories of the majority of carbohydrates; therefore, they induce a much lower daily consumption of food, in terms of quantity. The body burns stored fat more easily, just the ones you would like to dispose of, with the result that you lose more weight. The diet based on lipids keeps energy levels constant and avoids sudden increases in blood sugar, bypassing the highs and lows that occur when large quantities of carbohydrates are consumed. Maintaining a constant level of energy during the day allows you to be more dynamic and to feel less tired.

In addition to these benefits, the ketogenic diet has proved effective for:

- lose weight, especially in terms of fat mass;

- reduce blood sugar and insulin resistance, which frequently leads to the development of prediabetes and type 2 diabetes;

- reduce triglycerides;

- lower blood pressure; increase good cholesterol (HDL) and decrease bad cholesterol (LDL);

- improve brain function.

For Diabetics

A diet low in carbohydrates is also indicated for diabetics. Indeed, in the case of type 2 diabetes, it can radically change the situation, while in type 1 diabetes, it is particularly useful for keeping blood sugar under control.

However, always consult your doctor before embarking on a low-carb diet, especially if you have type 1 diabetes, because it is possible that you should immediately reduce the doses of the medications you take. Your doctor may also advise you to take a test, during which you will monitor your blood sugar levels and insulin dosage. The most common causes of ketoacidosis are type 1 diabetes and extreme fasting, which can lead to diabetic ketoacidosis and fasting ketoacidosis, respectively. However, ketoacidosis rarely occurs outside type 1 diabetes.

The proportions

Just like a Food Pyramid, the ketogenic plant-based diet is also based on the proportion of nutrients. It is indeed important to have the right balance of macronutrients to ensure that the body has the energy it needs and is not deficient in essential fats or proteins.

Chapter 4:

Shopping List for an Effective Plant-Based Diet

Basically, in a plant-based diet, you eat plants and only plants. There is an elimination of animal products and that includes dairy but don't be scared because this guide will help you make the change gradually without pressure.

There are many plant-based foods that people are not used to eating in their daily lives. These foods have hence fallen off the radar of most people and only the popular plant products come to mind when you think about a plant-based diet. Also, this is another factor that might put you off this diet because you think that there are only a handful of plant related products that you can eat. You are wrong because there is this a huge section of plants that are edible, delicious and you have no idea about them. For example, here is a list of plants products, some of which you may have heard but most of which would be unknown to you –

- Tofu
- Broccoli
- Tempeh
- Seitan
- Kale
- Quinoa
- Chia seeds (ground)
- Flaxseeds (ground)

- Walnuts
- Raw almonds
- Butter of raw almonds
- Black beans
- Hemp seeds
- Spirulina
- Organic soymilk
- Nutritional yeast

- Flourless sprouted bread
- Steel cut oats
- Brown rice

The ultimate plant-based diet is also known by the term "veganism" and although, some plant-based dieters do include certain animal products, the best and the healthiest option is going vegan.

What to avoid in a plant-based diet

Meat: All kinds of meat products such as fish, seafood, poultry, red meat, and even processed meat products are not allowed in a plant-based diet.

Eggs: You can't eat eggs, as it contains high cholesterol content.

Dairy: All forms of dairy products are not accepted in this diet. You have to avoid milk, yogurt, cream, cheese, buttermilk, and half-and-half.

Vegan replacements: Vegan replacements of meats and cheese are also not allowed. Such replacements contain high oil content, which is not acceptable in the plant-based diet.

Added fat: You have to say no to all kinds of added fats such as coconut oil, butter, margarine, and all other liquid oils.

Refined flours: Any flour that is not 100% in terms of whole wheat is not accepted. You can't use refined flours in your diet.

Added sugar: Any food item with added flavoring or sugar is not allowed. Along with that, you have to say no to energy bars, candy bars, cakes, cookies, and all other junk food options.

Beverages: In the category of beverages, you can't have soda or even fruit juices. Even the fruit juices with 100% purity are not allowed. At the same time, you are recommended to stay away from energy drinks, sports drinks, tea drinks, blended coffee, and other harmful beverages that contain flavorings or high-sugar content.

Chapter 5:

Tips on How to Resist Temptations, Control Craving and What to Do in Restaurants, or if Invited for a Dinner

One thing that I have heard so many people worry and stress about when beginning to adopt a vegan diet is that they will miss the meat, or they're worried about how to get the protein and iron. I've even had so many friends think they couldn't do it because they would miss meat so much and they were scared they wouldn't be able to keep it up over time. So whether you're just becoming a vegan now or you already are one, we're going to tell you how to start on this diet and how to stay on this diet. The one thing I recommend the most is if you're really worried about cutting meat from your diet, go slow. Also, if it helps, there are so many yummy alternatives to meat and you can find them at just about any supermarket which should make the switch even easier. Another thing to remind people is that once you begin adjusting to this diet, you will probably begin to crave meat less and less. Many people have said that they have been vegan for most of their lives and don't miss meat at all. Others say they feel bad for the meat eaters who are missing out on what plant based and vegans enjoy every day, from the great health benefits of the food to the wonderful flavors of the new foods in their diet.

You should also begin adding to your diet before taking things away. Familiarize yourself with how you prepare your new food, how it's stored, and the uses they have. With studying, you will see that many of your items can be used as multipurpose items. Olive oil is great for your skin and hair just as one example of how it can be used in a different way. You should start adding more vegan staples but keep in mind that you're both a vegan and ketogenic, not just one or the other. This means that there are certain things that ketogenic eat that vegans don't; like fish or meat for ketogenic; for vegans, most eat beans or potatoes and starchy foods but ketogenic usually avoid them because of the high carb content. So when adding things to your diet, keep in mind what you need to avoid and what will bring the most benefits to your new lifestyle.

Grow your own food. This one not everyone can do. Obviously, if you live in an apartment or are renting a house, you have to follow rules and wouldn't be able to do this one. But if you can, grow your own food. You could grow the food you eat and earn a deeper appreciation for your food and what's going in your body. You'll be able to see the work and effort it takes to provide yourself sustenance and you might even help other people try new things because the tastes are different. You can grow anything from vegetables to spices. The really cool thing though is if there's something you want to eat but can't find it anywhere, you can grow it yourself. Now, obviously, if you have to grow it, you won't get it when you want it because it would take weeks or months before it would be ready to eat. However, you will be able to have access to it which is a pretty cool thing to think about. If your garden got big enough, you could share with your finds and family and maybe they would be interested in eating healthier foods for themselves and their family because of your example.

Another surprising thing in this digital age is that you can have groceries delivered to you, even fresh ones in certain cases. This might help people who don't have vegan options near them. It will be easier for you to have it delivered especially if you live far away from the city or you're far from a place that actually carries what you need. Online shopping can also be a great way to try some new snacks as long as you're making sure it's not junk food or overly processed stuff that is going to make you gain a lot of weight. Look for options you know are good.

Remember, this is a journey. If you slip up, forgive and motivate yourself to do better so it won't happen again. If you're tired of the current options you're eating, find/keep trying new recipes and foods that you love. Keep looking around and exploring so that your knowledge keeps expanding. This can be a really fun way to make yourself happy and healthy and make sure that you accomplish the goals that you want to reach for yourself.

1) How to resist temptations

A fun way to get yourself used to this new lifestyle is to experiment with different recipes that sound good to you. You'll either realize that you like it and want to eat it again or maybe share it with the people around you if you live with others. Or maybe, instead, you'll be able to tell that it's something you don't like and wouldn't want to try again. Or maybe, it's just something you didn't like cooking. In that case, if you liked the dish but didn't like the work it took to prepare it, which happens to many people, that might lead you to a new restaurant that has the foods you can eat, and you might like how they prepare it. Once you begin experimenting and getting comfortable making the meals, it will become easier to adopt a new diet and find new foods that you like.

You can alter the recipes you already have and use on a daily basis too. If you eat meals with meat, make them plant based and then make them vegan before final making them ketogenic or Keto for short. You're still eating a meal that you already enjoy, it is just a different version of it. This can help you with your transition because it's just adapting things you're already used to. An example would be chili. Chili doesn't have to include meat at all, but if you really want it, try a meat substitute. Since beans aren't good for ketogenic because most of them are high in carbs, be sure to go through those carefully looking into the carb content and find a better option for that part of the diet as well. You could come up with an amazing recipe no one ever thought of before or you might be willing to try recipes that you wouldn't before this.

Getting support will help you be able to stick to your diet as well. Having people around that love you and support you can be a very big help during this transition. Family can be a big help when you're making such a drastic change. If you are not able to be around encouraging people, then be sure to find motivation and encourage yourself. Too many diets come with negativity and people making fun of others for trying something different. If this is what happens to you, I am sorry because no one deserves that at all and it can be very painful for someone to have to go through. The best thing you can do is ignore the hate and keep a positive attitude and remember what you're doing this for. You're doing this for you, not them, and you don't need their negativity. Ignore it and brush it off and stick to what you really want. I know it can be difficult but just remember you don't need to keep that negativity around you and you are stronger than they are. You are the one that lives your life and you should be happy. Remember this and just keep pushing through. I recommend a reward for you as well. For instance, if you managed to stay a vegan ketogenic for a month, reward yourself with something you've been wanting, like a new pair of shoes or a movie that you've wanted to see. The act of giving yourself a reward will send a positive vibe to your brain that will reinforce your healthy habits and help you to want to keep going on your journey.

Later, you feel guilty and ashamed which only hurts you and your progress as well as your emotional being. If you slip up, remember you are human. It can happen to anyone and there is no reason to feel guilty or ashamed. Slip-ups happen. The best thing we can do is to try again on the diet and try your best not to slip up. It is also important to note that slip-ups will probably happen in the first couple of days and if they do, it's alright. The important thing is that you're trying to better yourself and that you want to change. This is a good thing. Reminding yourself of that will help guide you because you will be able to understand that the effort you're putting forth is something to be proud of and one day you won't slip up at all.

2) How to control cravings

A good tip to start out is do not go cold turkey. No pun intended. When you go cold turkey without adequate preparation, you tend to be more likely to go back to eating meat and your old diet. Then you feel guilty and it can be a bad cycle. Removing it slowly over time is the best way to go about this because you're familiarizing your body to the new food and letting go of the old. Over time, you'll notice that you're craving meat less and the switch will become easier. A good example to go with is let's say you're trying to cut sweets out of your diet. So you remove anything with sugar in your house. Then you start to eat healthy for maybe a few hours or a day and you begin to get cravings. The problem with many people is that they get so hungry because they don't have the proper research about what to eat, and then they end up going on a binge or running out to the nearest place with cookies or they stay home, and binge eat. Now, you might think binging on healthy food is better but it's not. Binge eating is never healthy and can lead to eating disorders which are a bad thing.

3) What to do in restaurants

Make sure you stay informed. You need to make sure you've got good information going into this because that will help you know what you can and can't eat, or wear or use on your body when you visit a restaurant. Also, stay up to date on science and studies. People are still researching these diets and lifestyles to give people the correct information. If you stay up to date, you'll be able to see the new information too.

If you feel like you can't do it, remind yourself why you decided to do this in the first place. Remind yourself of the facts. Watch videos online or read studies. They say it's harder to slip when you see the facts presented to you and you're watching the consequences of eating meat.

Finding new items and recipes can be a fun and exciting adventure and a great way to keep yourself on track. We can always learn new things and for a lot of people, going on little adventures can be a lot of fun. Get out and about and see what vegan things you can find around you.

Find inspiration. There are so many celebrities that have taken up the cause and so many other people as well. Doctors, lawyers, teachers; there are so many people now that have joined the vegan move. There are also many organizations that have taken up the movement as well. Be careful with these organizations though and make sure they are on the up and up. Studies have shown that some organizations kill more animals than they save. Or some don't follow the ideas you have for yourself. You need to make sure that you find inspiration that is going to help you. Thanks to social media, you can even be connected to hundreds of thousands of people that have the same lifestyle and desires to help animals as you do. You can ask questions and learn everything you can about the vegan lifestyle. As with anything on social media though, you need to be careful as there are dangers beyond bad advice as some people simply can't be trusted so you'll need to be careful that you don't get hurt.

As you adapt to this lifestyle more and more, you should be able to stay on it much easier. Some good tips for maintaining your vegan lifestyle is if you like to eat out, it's like we said it can be difficult with your eating needs. So find out in advance where you can and can't go.

4) What to do when invited for dinner

You can be at a dinner with a few friends and they want to share an appetizer and you think one won't hurt, or they want to drink so you figure one drink won't have too many carbs or something along those lines. A quick tip though; a lot of drinks do have carbs and on a ketogenic diet, it is really not recommended because you'll bust straight through your numbers. Some people even give in to the peer pressure because their friends get upset that someone is not eating like the rest of them. Ignore the peer pressure and do what you want to do. You don't have to answer to anyone but yourself.

Have special food you can take with you when you leave your house. More and more places are trying to accommodate people's needs but some just don't have everything that you are able to eat because your diet can be a little bit restrictive. This is really going to help you keep yourself from being tempted by other's influence or choices or if a place you're at can't meet the needs of your diet. When you're out at social situations, it can be tempting to get out of your diet or eat foods you know you shouldn't. We have all been there.

Offer to make dinner for your friends or ask if you can make some vegan dishes to a dinner or party. More often than not, you will see that they're really interested in what you have to say and that they will love how amazing your food tastes. They may even opt to go vegan themselves! A perfect example is let's say all your meat-eater friends are having a dinner party and want you to bring a Soups and stew. Okay, easy peas. Make them some vegan Keto zucchini brownies, or some vegan Keto cupcakes and watch them fall in love. I bet you won't even be able to tell that there are healthy vegetables in there and your friends will fall in love.

Make your lifestyle the new norm. Everyone thinks that meat-eating is the norm; switch what it means. Now, this doesn't mean getting in people's faces and being rude or abrupt. Be kind and polite. It can be hard for people to change and some people are just blissfully unaware. Be happy in the knowledge that you're making a difference and try to feel compassionate to people no matter what choices they make. If you are content with who you are, it is more likely that people will be open to talking to you about this. They could even begin questioning their own choices. I have known so many people that have gotten upset and hurt when vegans challenged them and pushed too far. But by simply being an awesome and secure person who's happy in their choices, you'll probably begin to see that your friends want to come to you because they see you so happy and want to know what your secret is.

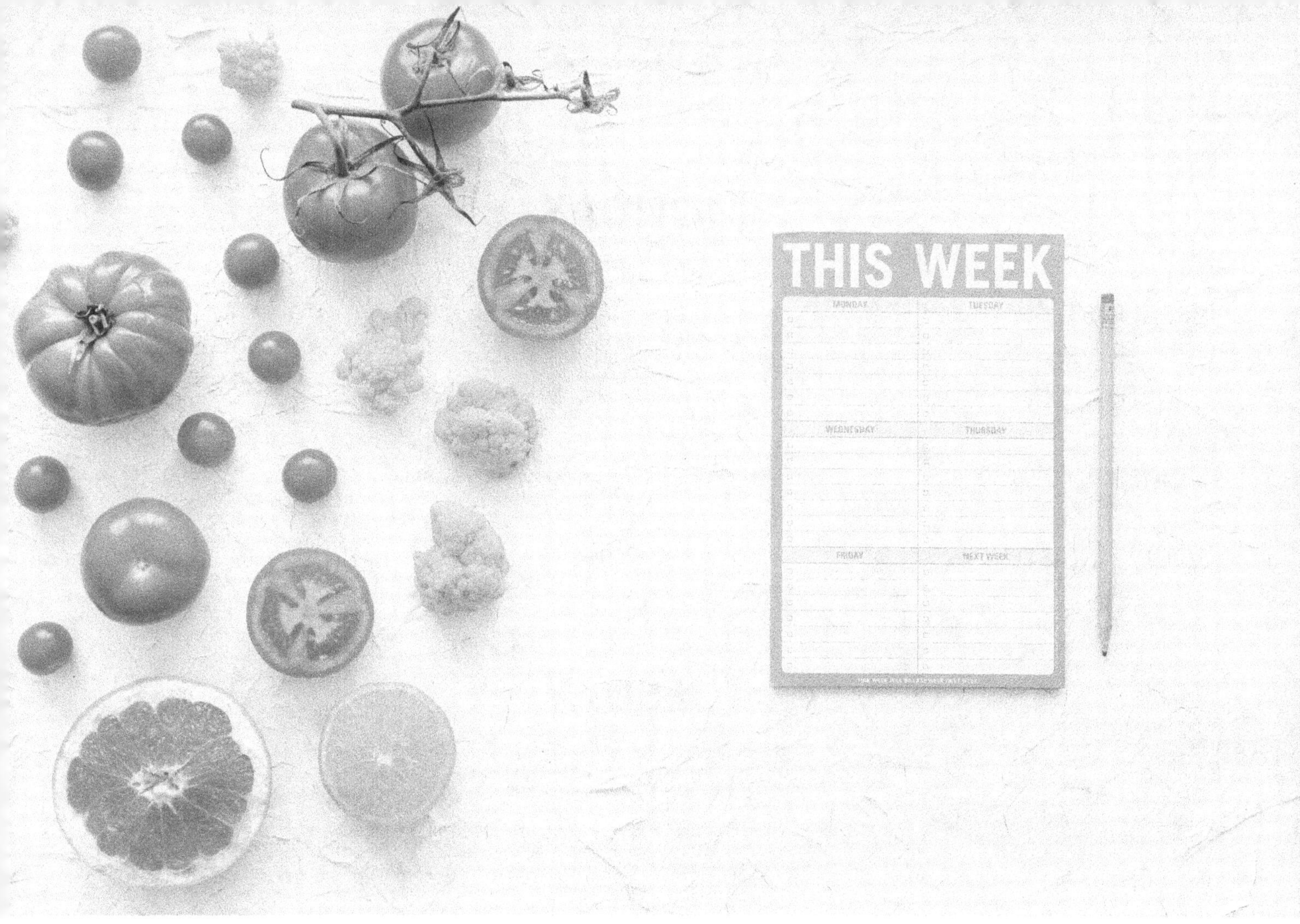

Chapter 6:

Weekly Plan

So how do you make the plant based-Keto diet work for you? In this chapter, you will see a 7-day meal plan that will show you how to make the plant based-Keto diet work for you. Each day is designed to provide you with a plant based-Keto meal that is supporting your weight loss efforts.

MONDAY

BREAKFAST:	Flaxseed Porridge
LUNCH:	Zucchini & Lemon Salad
DINNER:	Tomato Gazpacho
SOUPS AND STEWS:	White Bean & Spinach Soup

TUESDAY

BREAKFAST:	Avocado & Strawberry Bowl
LUNCH:	Red Pepper & Broccoli Salad
DINNER:	Grilled Eggplant Steaks
SOUPS AND STEWS:	Thai Squash Soup

WEDNESDAY

BREAKFAST:	Coconut & Strawberry Bars
LUNCH:	Mediterranean Wrap
DINNER:	Sushi Bowl
SOUPS AND STEWS:	Quinoa with Nectarine Slaw

THURSDAY

BREAKFAST:	Green Mango Smoothie
LUNCH:	Olive & Fennel Salad
DINNER:	Cauliflower Steaks
SOUPS AND STEWS:	Red Lentil Soup

FRIDAY

BREAKFAST:	Kiwi Slushie
LUNCH:	Summer Chickpea Salad
DINNER:	Fried Pineapple Rice
SOUPS AND STEWS:	Black Eyed Peas Stew

SATURDAY

BREAKFAST:	Flaxseed Pancakes
LUNCH:	Edamame Salad
DINNER:	Tofu Poke
SOUPS AND STEWS:	Red Lentil Soup

SUNDAY

BREAKFAST:	Pumpkin Chia Smoothie
LUNCH:	Fruity Kale Salad
DINNER:	Fried Pineapple Rice
SOUPS AND STEWS:	Cabbage & Beet Stew

Each day is laid out with a breakfast option, a lunch option, a dinner option, as well as a snack or side dish. This is a basic example of a 7-day meal plan with the Plant based-keto diet.

Tips to incorporate into your new Plant-Based-Keto diet Plan

The number one tip that I could give you is that coconut is king. What this means is that coconut products become your best friend while on the plant based-keto diet. They are low in carbs and provide several ways to incorporate them into your life. Coconut is as great as creams, milks and butters. It adds to the flavor of your meals and coconut milk has been known to lower your blood pressure, improving your cholesterol and is so nourishing. You can add coconut to just about anything, such as smoothies, curries, and even yogurts.

The second tip that will help you with your plant based-keto diet is that since oatmeal is high in carbs, a great alternative is chia seeds. They are very low on the net carb count due to their higher fiber content. Chia seeds absorb the flavor of your food. That makes them a very flexible ingredient for many types of meals. Because they expand and become sort of like jelly, this makes them an excellent breakfast food.

A good way to use chia seeds is to place 50 g of chia seeds into a bowl with water and placing it in the fridge till the next day. Bring it out in the morning and enjoy a great, nutritious, low carb breakfast. Alternatively, you can use milk instead of water, or yogurt.

Adding other things to spice up the flavor is going to be necessary since chia seeds are quite bland on their own. So, use some coconut milk, cinnamon, flax seeds, almonds, coconut cream, yogurt, fruit and any number of ingredients and herbs to flavor your breakfast chia seeds.

A long time ago, the nutritional gods told us that oil was not our friend. But that has all changed with the plant based-keto diet. Tip number three is that oil is your new best friend. By using ketones for your fuel, you can now enjoy oils as a healthy, tasty, and very flavorful fuel source. It is versatile while also being easy. You should keep a variety of oils on hand for all your cooking and oil needs. Drizzle them over vegetables and enjoy the transformation of flavors. Using oils helps you to be more flexible with your meal plan. So, add more oils and don't worry about your carb count since they are low in carbs. Include oils such as monounsaturated and polyunsaturated fats.

- Flaxseed oil
- Coconut oil
- Macadamia oil
- Avocado oil
- Olive oil

Avoid oils that are high in trans-fat, heavily processed, and containing any unnatural flavoring.

- Canola oil
- Soybean oil
- Cottonseed oil
- Safflower oil
- Sunflower oil

Tip number four is to incorporate many different types of foods into your plant based-keto diet. Make sure you include lots of low carb vegetables such as spinach, broccoli, mushrooms, and asparagus. You also want to have a variety of nuts and seeds as well as multivitamins.

FAQS to know before you start the Plant Based-Keto diet

The most important FAQ that you need to know before starting the Keto diet with a plant-based lifestyle is that it is not meant for long-term use. Keto is scientifically proven to show non-beneficial long-term results. This does not mean that you cannot correct your unhealthy lifestyle choices with the Keto diet. It does mean that consulting a doctor before attempting to change to the plant based-keto diet is a necessary step in ensuring that you are properly following it and you are not doing any harm to your system. Using it intermittently is ok. However, do not use it permanently. Cycling in and out of ketosis is your best option when using the keto diet.

When following the plant-based lifestyle, you should use whole foods, and not any canned vegetables. The vegetables in a can are not nutritionally sound options and can be less nutritious than you know. The whole food items will help you hit your goals on caloric intake. They also are very rich in slow-digesting carbs that can help maintain energy levels in the long run. Avoid processed foods since they are stripped of many of the positive nutrients that you need to sustain a healthy lifestyle. Also, staying away from sugars and carbs is your best bet, especially since you are combining Keto with plant basedism. These nutrients that are missing in the processed foods are needed for the blocking of sugar from being absorbed into your bloodstream too quickly. So, avoid these all together.

Make sure you follow up on your vitamins and minerals with some blood work with your doctor. Often times, plant based-keto dieters will miss important nutrients, minerals, and vitamins that are needed in their bodies. Three of the major ones that are usually lacking, but highly needed are iron, Omega-3 fatty acids, and B12.

B12 is mostly found in heme-iron, which is mostly found in animal products. Fish is loaded with Omega-3, making it a great source option. However, on the plant based-keto diet, fish is out of the question. So, follow our recommendations for gaining all the Omega-3 you can get. Zinc as well as calcium, and Vitamin D, along with magnesium are all important nutrients, vitamins, and minerals that are usually lacking in those who are plant based.

Due to the conflicting recommended food options in the plant based-keto diet, you should talk with a dietitian or nutritionist before starting this diet plan. This will ensure that you are following the diet as recommended by the doctors and nutritionists. It also ensures that you are getting the necessary nutrients, vitamins, and minerals you need for optimal health.

Chapter 7:

Breakfast Recipes

VEGETABLE HASH

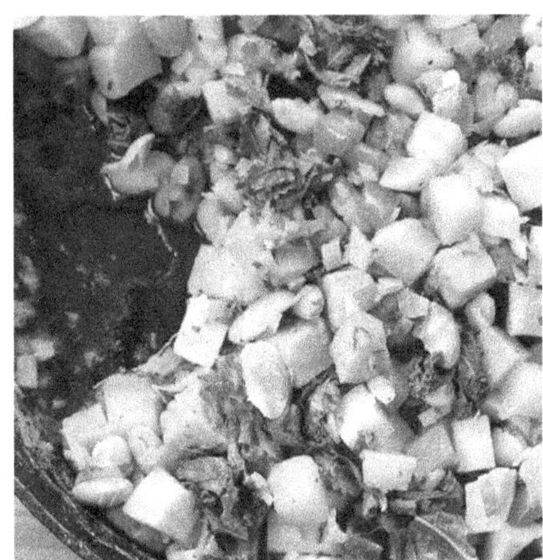

Serves: 4
Time: 35 Minutes

Calories: 273
Protein: 9 Grams
Fat: 11 Grams
Carbs: 39 Grams

INGREDIENTS:

- 1 Tablespoon Sage Leaves, Chopped
- 1 Bell Pepper, Diced
- 3 Cloves Garlic, Minced
- 1 Onion, Diced
- 3 Tablespoons Olive Oil
- 3 Red Potatoes, Diced
- 15 Ounces Black Beans, Canned
- 1 Tablespoon Parsley, Chopped
- 2 Cups Swiss Chard, Chopped
- Sea Salt & Black Pepper to Taste

DIRECTIONS:

1. Start by cooking your potato, garlic and onion in a skillet with your oil. This will take twenty minutes.

2. Add in your Swiss chard and beans, cooking for three more minutes.

3. Season

Interesting Facts: Potatoes are a great starchy source of potassium and protein. They are pretty inexpensive if you are one that is watching their budget. Bonus: Very heart healthy!

FLAXSEED PANCAKES

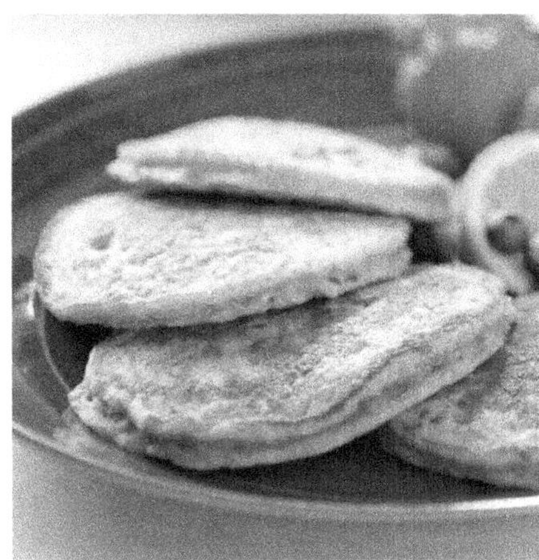

Serves: 1
Time: 15 Minutes

Calories: 309
Protein: 13.4 Grams
Fat: 27.1 Grams
Carbs: 5 Grams

INGREDIENTS:

- 3 Tablespoons Water
- 2 Tablespoons Flaxseeds
- Pinch Sea Salt
- 1 ½ Tablespoons Coconut Oil
- ½ Scoop Vanilla Vegan Powder
- ¼ Teaspoon Baking Powder

DIRECTIONS:

1. Mix a tablespoon of flaxseeds with water, and then mix in your oil.

2. Mix your baking powder, protein powder, flax seed and salt together in a bowl.

3. Heat a nonstick pan over medium heat containing ingredients.

4. Scoop batter into your pan, cooking for five minutes. Flip cooking for two minutes on the other side. Repeat until you've finished all your batter.

Interesting Facts: Flaxseeds: These guys are awesome add-ins to most plant-based meals since they can be ground up and added to things such as cookies, muffins, bread, cereal, oatmeal, and smoothies. They are packed with B vitamins, zinc, magnesium, and protein. Bonus: They aid in digestion and assist with suppressing appetite, which aids in weight loss!

AVOCADO BREAKFAST BOWL

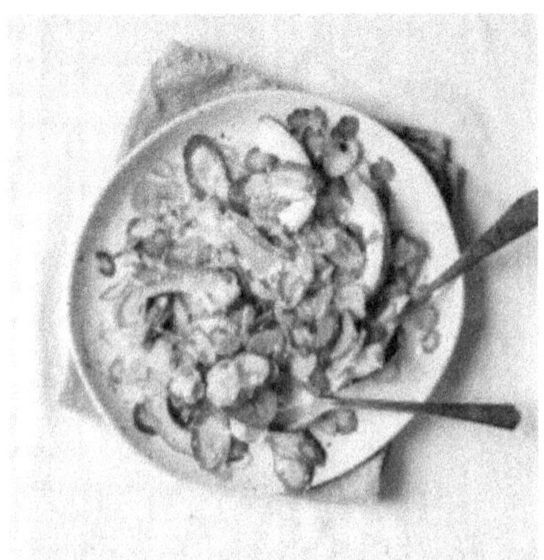

Serves:	1
Time:	5 Minutes
Calories:	562
Protein:	8 Grams
Fat:	52 Grams
Carbs:	7 Grams

INGREDIENTS:

- 2 Tablespoons Tahini
- 1 Carrot, Shredded
- 1 Avocado, Halved & Pit Removed

SAUCE:

- Sea Salt to Taste
- ¼ Cup Olive Oil
- 1 Teaspoon Ginger, Fresh & Grated
- 1 Tablespoon Poppy Seeds
- ¼ Cup Lemon Juice

DIRECTIONS:

1. Mix all other ingredients together.

2. Drizzle your sauce over your bowl before serving.

Interesting Facts: Avocado Oil: Avocados themselves are ranked within the top five of the healthiest foods on the planet, so you know that the oil that is produced from them is too. It is loaded with healthy fats and essential fatty acids. Like race bran oil it is perfect to cook with as well! Bonus: Helps in the prevention of diabetes and lowers cholesterol levels.

COCONUT & STRAWBERRY BARS

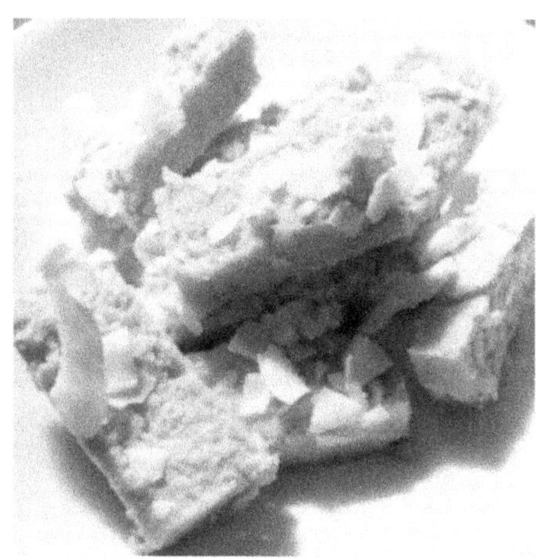

Serves: 2
Time: 4 Hours 10 Minutes

Calories: 294
Protein: 3 Grams
Fat: 28 Grams
Carbs: 4 Grams

INGREDIENTS:

- 1 Tablespoon Coconut Oil
- 1 Cup Strawberries, Chopped
- 16 Ounces Coconut Butter, Melted
- 1 Teaspoon Stevia
- ¼ Cup Coconut Flakes, Unsweetened

DIRECTIONS:

1. Mix your stevia, oil, and butter together, transferring it to a prepared baking dish.

2. Add your strawberries and coconut, and then refrigerate for four hours. Chop into bars.

Interesting Facts: Coconut Oil: Coconut oil is full of healthy fats that are absorbed easily in the human body. It is a go-to when it comes to Vegan cooking since it is a great substitute for butter and vegetable oils. It can also be used topically, in treating hair and skin. Bonus: Contains fatty acids that aid in weight loss. Double Bonus: Strengthens the immune system.

SPICY HASH BROWNS

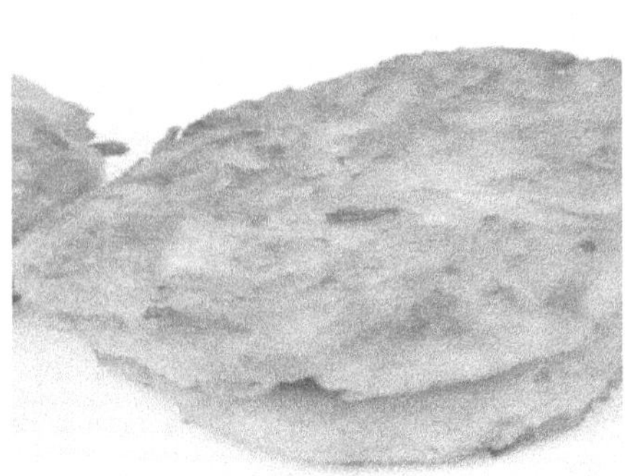

Serves:	5
Time:	45 Minutes
Calories:	227
Protein:	3.9 Grams
Fat:	5.7 Grams
Carbs:	41.3 Grams

INGREDIENTS:

- 1 Teaspoon Paprika
- ¼ Teaspoon Red Pepper
- ¾ Teaspoon Chili Powder
- 2 Tablespoons Olive Oil
- 6 ½ Cups Potatoes, Diced
- Sea Salt & Black Pepper to Taste

DIRECTIONS:

1. Start by heating your oven to 400, and then get out a large bowl.

2. Mix together your olive oil, chili powder, red peppers, salt, black pepper, and paprika. Stir well.

3. Coat your potatoes in the mixture, and then arrange your potatoes on a baking sheet in a single layer

4. Bake for about thirty minutes.

Interesting Facts: Potatoes are a great starchy source of potassium and protein. They are pretty inexpensive if you are one that is watching their budget. Bonus: Very heart healthy!

CANTALOUPE SMOOTHIE BOWL

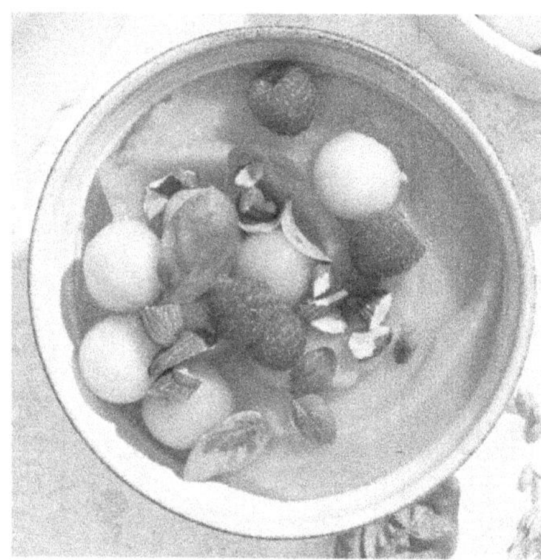

Serves: 2
Time: 5 Minutes

Calories: 135
Protein: 3 Grams
Fat: 1 Gram
Carbs: 32 Grams

INGREDIENTS:

- ¾ Cup carrot Juice
- 4 Cps Cantaloupe, Frozen & Cubed
- Mellon Balls or Berries to Serve
- Pinch Sea Salt

DIRECTIONS:

1. Blend everything together until smooth.

Interesting Facts: These guys are a delectable treat that is easily incorporated into many dishes. They are packed with antioxidants and Vitamin C. Bonus: Blueberries have been proven to promote eye health and slow macular degeneration.

FLAXSEED PORRIDGE

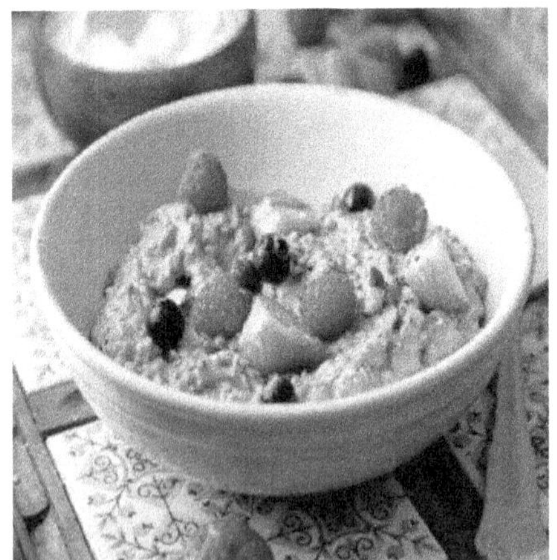

Serves:	2
Time:	15 Minutes
Calories:	405
Protein:	10 Grams
Fat:	34 Grams
Carbs:	12 Grams

INGREDIENTS:

- 1 Cup Almond Milk
- 1 Teaspoon Cinnamon
- ¼ Cup Coconut Flour
- ¼ Cup Ground Flaxseed
- 10 Drops Stevia
- 1 Teaspoon Vanilla Extract, Pure
- Pinch Sea Salt
- 1 Ounces Coconut, Shaved for Garnish
- 2 Ounces Blueberries for Garnish
- 2 Tablespoons Almond Butter for Garnish
- 2 Tablespoons Pumpkin Seeds for Garnish

DIRECTIONS:

1. Heat your almond milk in a saucepan using low heat, and whisk your coconut flour, salt, cinnamon and flaxseed together.

2. Add in your stevia and vanilla once it's bubbling

3. Remove it from heat, mixing all of your ingredients together.

4. Garnish with blueberries, coconut, pumpkin seeds and almonds before serving.

Interesting Facts: Flaxseeds: These guys are awesome add-ins to most plant-based meals since they can be ground up and added to things such as cookies, muffins, bread, cereal, oatmeal, and smoothies. They are packed with B vitamins, zinc, magnesium, and protein. Bonus: They aid in digestion and assist with suppressing appetite, which aids in weight loss!

BERRY & CAULIFLOWER SMOOTHIE

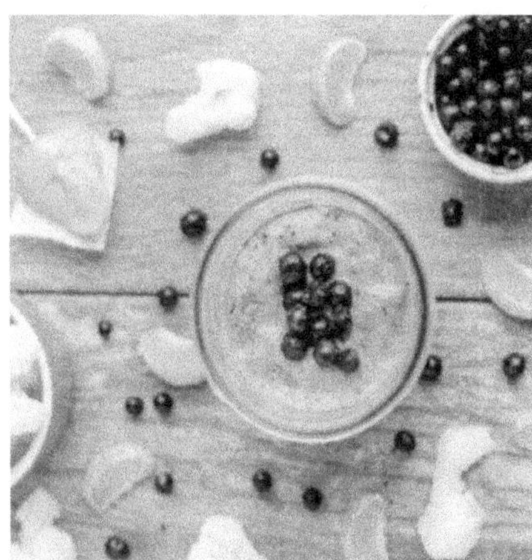

Serves:	2
Time:	10 Minutes
Calories:	149
Protein:	3 Grams
Fat:	3 Grams
Carbs:	29 Grams

INGREDIENTS:

- 1 Cup Riced Cauliflower, Frozen

- 1 Cup Banana, Sliced & Frozen

- ½ Cup Mixed Berries, Frozen

- 2 Cups Almond Milk, Unsweetened

- 2 Teaspoons Maple syrup, Pure & Optional

DIRECTIONS:

1. Blend until mixed well.

Interesting Facts: This vegetable is an extremely high source of vitamin A, vitamin B1, B2 and B3. It has even been said that it can be used as a stress reliever!

QUINOA & CHOCOLATE BOWL

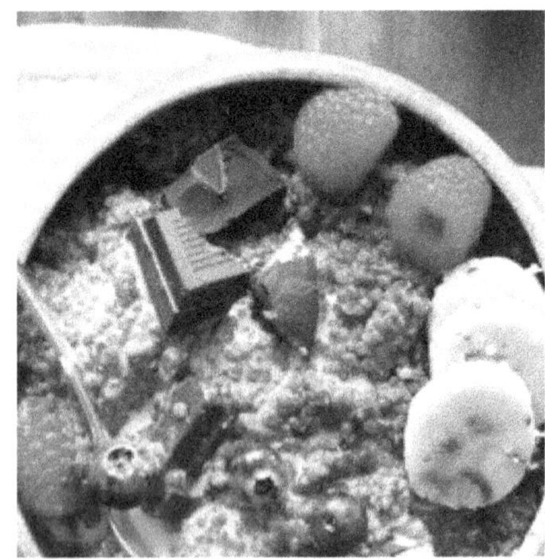

Serves: 2
Time: 35 Minutes

Calories: 392
Protein: 12 Grams
Fat: 19 Grams
Carbs: 49 Grams

INGREDIENTS:

- 1 Cup Quinoa
- 1 Cup Almond Milk, Unsweetened
- 1 Teaspoon Cinnamon
- 1 Banana
- 1 Cup Water
- 2-3 Tablespoons Cocoa Powder, Unsweetened
- 2 Tablespoons Almond Butter
- 1 Tablespoon Chia Seeds, Ground
- 2 Tablespoons Walnuts, Optional
- ¼ Cup Raspberries, Fresh

DIRECTIONS:

1. Place your cinnamon, milk, water and quinoa in a pot, bringing it to a boil before turning it down to low heat to simmer. Cover, simmering for twenty-five to thirty minutes.

2. Puree your banana, mixing in your almond butter, flaxseed and cocoa powder.

3. Scoop a cup of quinoa into a bowl, and then top with pudding, raspberries and walnuts if you're using them before serving.

Interesting Facts: _Cinnamon:_ This spice is an absolute powerhouse and is considered one of the healthiest, beneficial spices on the plant. It's widely known for its medicinal properties. This spice is loaded with powerful antioxidants and is popular for its anti-inflammatory properties. It can reduce heart disease and lower blood sugar levels.

FLAXSEED & BLUEBERRY PORRIDGE

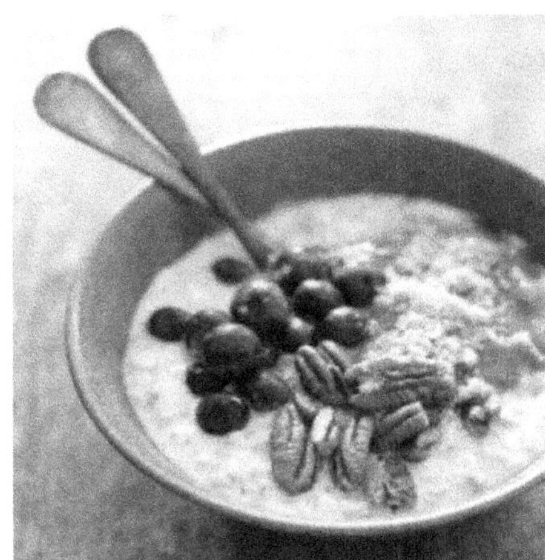

Serves: 2

Calories: 405
Protein: 10 Grams
Fat: 34 Grams
Carbs: 12 Grams

INGREDIENTS:

- 1 Cup Almond Milk
- ¼ Cup Coconut Flour
- 1 Teaspoon Cinnamon
- ¼ Cup Flaxseed, Ground

- 1 Teaspoon Vanilla Extract
- 10 Drops Stevia
- Pinch Sea Salt

GARNISH:

- 1 Ounces Coconut, Shaved
- 2 Tablespoon Pumpkin Seeds

- 2 Tablespoons Almond Butter
- 2 Ounces Blueberries

DIRECTIONS:

1. Over low heat, whisking in your coconut flour, salt, cinnamon and flaxseed

2. Once it bubbles, add in your vanilla and stevia

3. Remove from heat, garnishing as desired.

Interesting Facts: Pumpkin seeds are popularly known as a yummy snack, and can also be easily incorporated into soups, yogurt, salads, and more! They are loaded with iron, Vitamins C, E, and K, and essential omega-3s.

GREEN MANGO SMOOTHIE

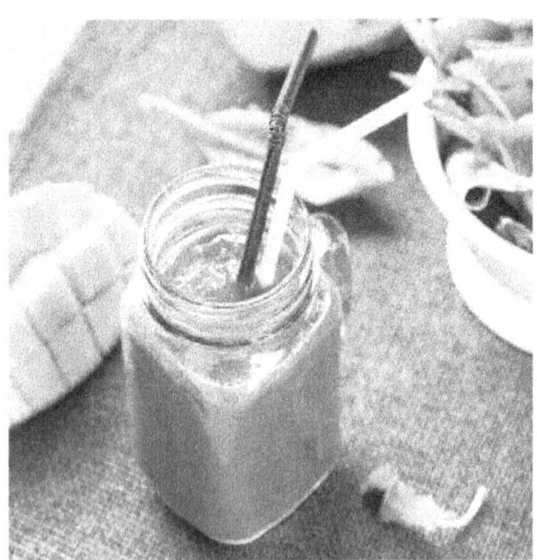

Serves:	1
Time:	5 Minutes
Calories:	417
Protein:	7.2 Grams
Fat:	2.8 Grams
Carbs:	102.8 Grams

INGREDIENTS:

- 2 Cups Spinach

- 1-2 Cups Coconut Water

- 2 Mangos, Ripe, Peeled & Diced

DIRECTIONS:

1. Blend everything together until smooth.

Interesting Facts: Mangos contain 50% of the daily Vitamin C you should consume which aid in bone and immune health.

EGGPLANT HASH BROWNS

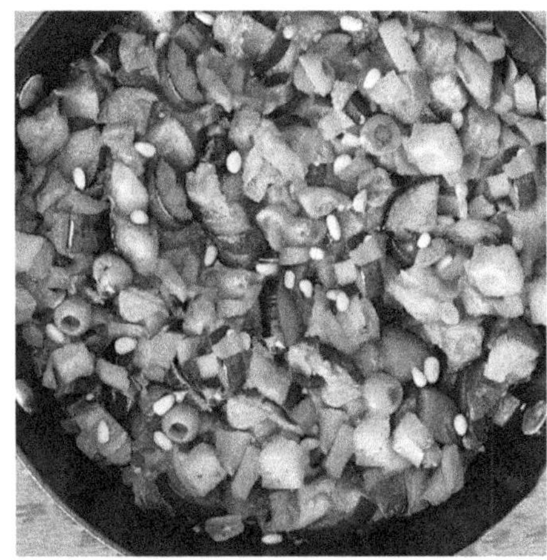

Serves: 8
Time: 20 Minutes

Calories: 100
Protein: 2.42 Grams
Fat: 6.4 Grams
Carbs: 8 Grams

INGREDIENTS:

- 1 Eggplant, Peeled, Cubed & Salted
- 2 Tablespoons Coconut Oil
- 1 Red Onion, Diced
- 2 Red Bell Peppers, Seeded & Diced
- 4 Cloves Garlic, Minced
- ¼ Cup Almonds, Slivered & Toasted
- ¼ Cup Mint Leaves, Fresh
- ½ Cup Sundried Tomatoes, Drained & Chopped
- ½ Teaspoon Coriander Seeds
- ¼ Teaspoon Cayenne Pepper
- ½ Teaspoon Cinnamon
- Sea Salt & Black Pepper to Taste

DIRECTIONS:

1. Start by heating oil in a skillet, searing your bell pepper and eggplant, cooking for three minutes. Make sure to stir occasionally.

2. Add in your onion and garlic, cooking for two minutes.

3. Toss in your mint leaves, almonds and tomatoes. Make sure to heat all the way through, and then add in the rest of your ingredients.

Interesting Facts: Eggplant has a variety of vital vitamins and minerals within it's compound. It is high in folic acid, vitamin C, manganese and vitamin K. It aids weight lose and cognitive function. Eggplant is a great meat replacement in a lasagna!

COCONUT & STRAWBERRY SMOOTHIE

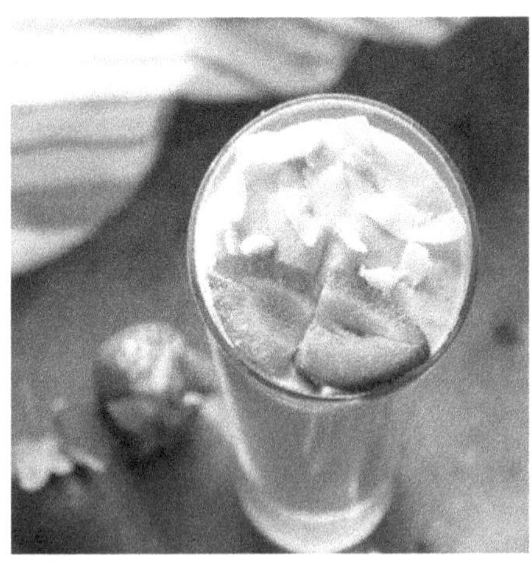

Serves: 1
Time: 10 Minutes

Calories: 278
Protein: 14 Grams
Fat: 2 Grams
Carbs: 57 Grams

INGREDIENTS:

- 1 Cup Strawberries, Frozen & Thawed Slightly
- 1 Ripe Banana, Sliced & Frozen
- ½ Cup Coconut Milk, Light
- ½ Cup Greek Yogurt, Plain
- 1 Tablespoon Chia Seeds
- 1 Teaspoon Lime juice, Fresh
- 4 Ice Cubes

DIRECTIONS:

1. Blend everything.

Interesting Facts: Coconut oil is full of healthy fats that are absorbed easily in the human body. It is a go-to when it comes to Vegan cooking since it is a great substitute for butter and vegetable oils. It can also be used topically, in treating hair and skin. Bonus: Contains fatty acids that aid in weight loss. Double Bonus: Strengthens the immune system.

KIWI SLUSHIE

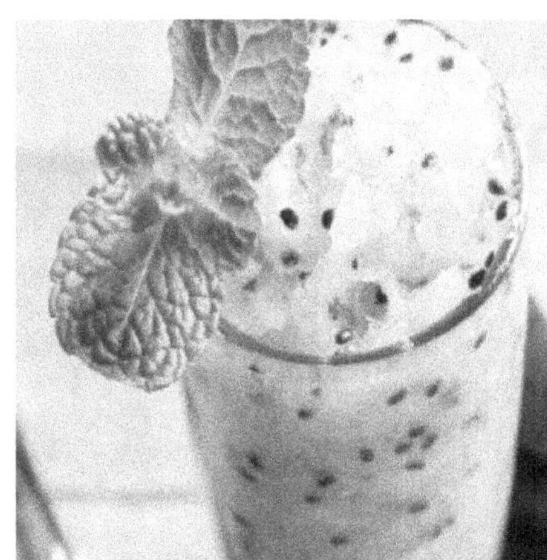

Serves:	2
Time:	5 Minutes
Calories:	42.1
Protein:	0.8 Grams
Fat:	0.4 Grams
Carbs:	10.1 Grams

INGREDIENTS:

- 18 Chocolate Tea Ice Cubes

- 1 Cup Vanilla Rice Milk

- 2 Ripe Kiwi Fruits, Sliced & Frozen

DIRECTIONS:

1. Blend everything together until smooth.

Interesting Facts: This tart fruit is loaded with Vitamins E and C, along with many types of antioxidants. They are loaded with fiber and have a low-calorie count, which makes them a guilt-free snack. Bonus: Promote eye health. Double Bonus: Lowers the chances of cancer. Triple Bonus: Aids in weight loss!

PUMPKIN CHIA SMOOTHIE

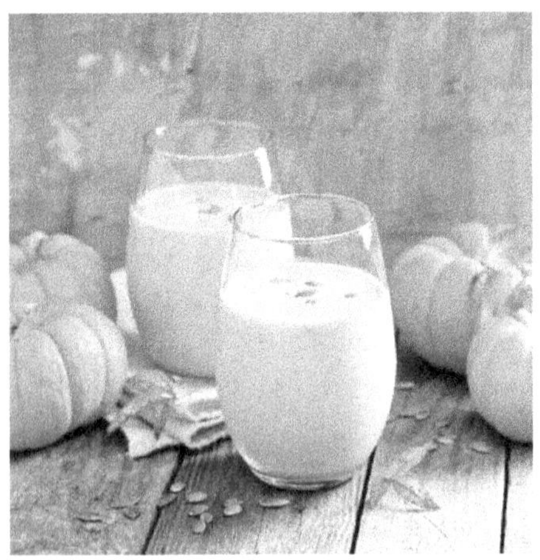

Serves:	1
Time:	5 Minutes
Calories:	726
Protein:	5.5 Grams
Fat:	69.8 Grams
Carbs:	15 Grams

INGREDIENTS:

- 3 Tablespoons Pumpkin Puree
- 1 Tablespoon MCT Oil
- ¾ Cup Coconut Milk, Full Fat
- ½ Avocado, Fresh
- 1 Teaspoon Vanilla, Pure
- ½ Teaspoon Pumpkin Pie Spice

DIRECTIONS:

1. Combine all ingredients together until blended.

Interesting Facts: Chia seeds are widely known to the vegan world and can be sprinkled on just about anything and everything. They are an amazing source of calcium, fiber, protein, and Vitamin C. Add them to your smoothies, breakfast meals and clean eating bowls for an extra bang!

BREAKFAST CEREAL

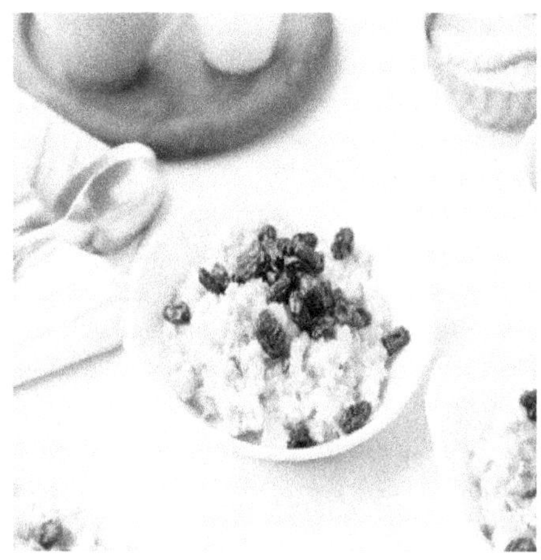

Serves: 6
Time: 45 Minutes

Calories: 160
Protein: 3 Grams
Fat: 1.5 Grams
Carbs: 34 Grams

INGREDIENTS:

- ¼ Tablespoon Butter
- 2 ¼ Cups Water
- Honey to Taste
- 1 Teaspoon Cinnamon
- 1 Cup Brown Rice, Uncooked
- ½ Cup Raisins, Seedless

DIRECTIONS:

1. Start by combining your cinnamon, raisins, rice, and butter in a saucepan before adding in your water. While covered for forty minutes, Fluff with a fork.

2. Serve with honey.

Interesting Facts: This spice is an absolute powerhouse and is considered one of the healthiest, beneficial spices on the plant. It's widely known for its medicinal properties. This spice is loaded with powerful antioxidants and is popular for its anti-inflammatory properties. It can reduce heart disease and lower blood sugar levels.

WALNUT PORRIDGE

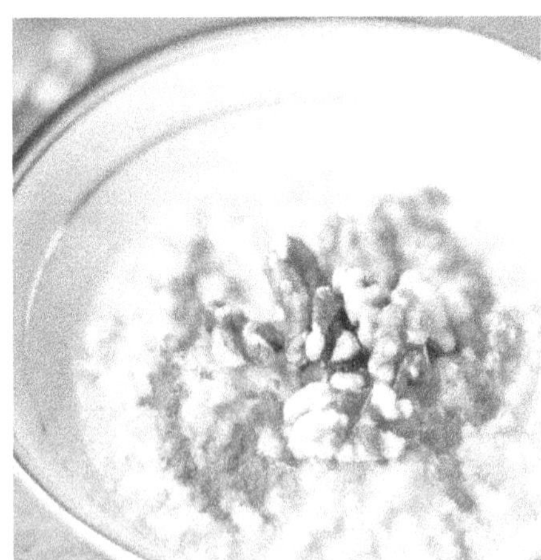

Serves:	2
Time:	25 Minutes
Calories:	312
Protein:	7 Grams
Fat:	18 Grams
Carbs:	35 Grams

INGREDIENTS:

- 1 ½ Cups Water
- ½ Cup Coconut Milk, Unsweetened
- 1 Cup Teff, Whole Grain
- ½ Teaspoon Cardamom, Ground
- 1 Teaspoon Sea Salt, Fine
- ¼ Cup Walnuts, Chopped
- 1 Tablespoon Maple Syrup, Pure

DIRECTIONS:

1. Start by combining your coconut oil and water, bringing it to a boil before stirring in your teff.

2. Add the cardamom, and then allow it to simmer for twenty minutes.

3. Mix in your walnuts and maple syrup before serving.

Interesting Facts: Walnuts have been proven to boost your metabolism, regulate sleep, assist in clear skin, heart function and bone health.

CHIA SEED SMOOTHIE

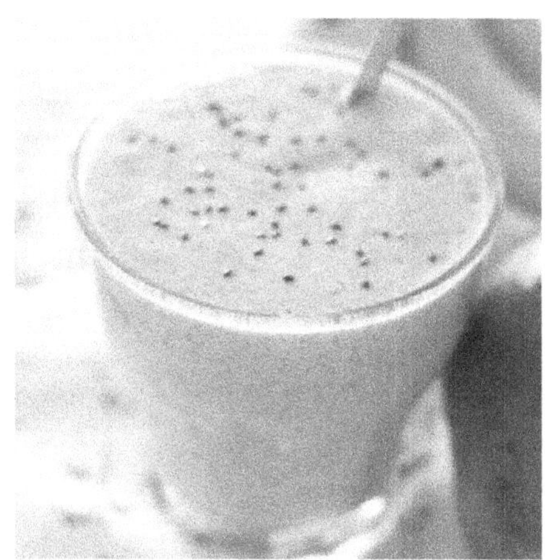

Serves: 3
Time: 5 Minutes

Calories: 477
Protein: 8 Grams
Fat: 29 Grams
Carbs: 57 Grams

INGREDIENTS:

- ¼ Teaspoon Cinnamon
- 1 Tablespoon Ginger, Fresh & Grated
- Pinch Cardamom
- 1 Tablespoon Chia Seeds
- 2 Medjool Dates, Pitted
- 1 Cup Alfalfa Sprouts
- 1 Cup Water
- 1 Banana
- ½ Cup Coconut Milk, Unsweetened

DIRECTIONS:

1. Blend everything together until smooth.

Interesting Facts: Chia seeds are widely known to the vegan world and can be sprinkled on just about anything and everything. They are an amazing source of calcium, fiber, protein, and Vitamin C. Add them to your smoothies, breakfast meals and clean eating bowls for an extra bang!

AVOCADO & STRAWBERRY BOWL

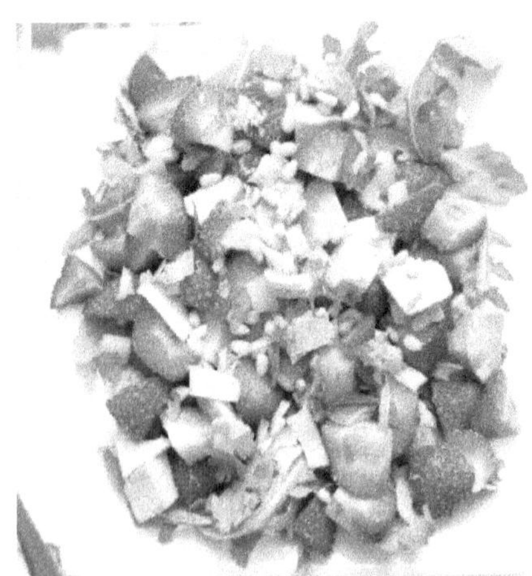

Serves: 1

Calories: 140
Protein: 2 Grams
Fat: 10 Grams
Carbs: 5 Grams

INGREDIENTS:

- 1 Cup Strawberries
- 1 Cup Avocado, Peeled & Pitted
- 1 Teaspoon Lime
- Stevia to Taste
- Pinch Sea Salt

DIRECTIONS:

1. Blend all ingredients until smooth.

Interesting Facts: Avocados themselves are ranked within the top five of the healthiest foods on the planet, so you know that the oil that is produced from them is too. It is loaded with healthy fats and essential fatty acids. Like race bran oil it is perfect to cook with as well! Bonus: Helps in the prevention of diabetes and lowers cholesterol levels.

MANGO SMOOTHIE

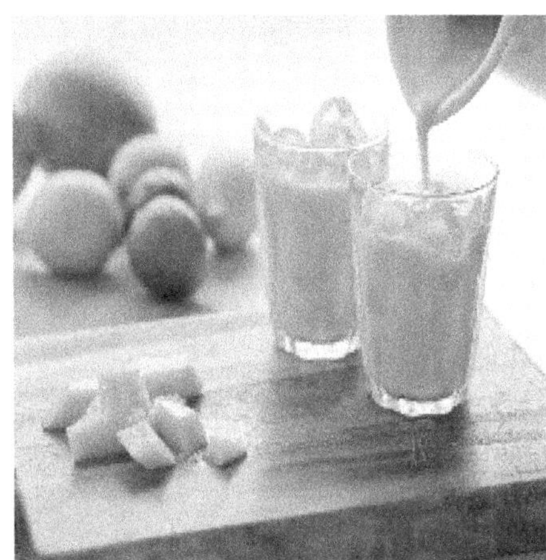

Serves: 3
Time: 5 Minutes

Calories: 376
Protein: 5 Grams
Fat: 2 Grams
Carbs: 95 Grams

INGREDIENTS:

- 1 Carrot, Peeled & Chopped
- 1 Cup Strawberries
- 1 Cup Water
- 1 Cup Peaches, Chopped
- 1 Banana, Frozen & sliced
- 1 Cup Mango, Chopped

DIRECTIONS:

1. Blend everything together until smooth.

Interesting Facts: Mangos contain 50% of the daily Vitamin C you should consume which aid in bone and immune health.

GRANOLA

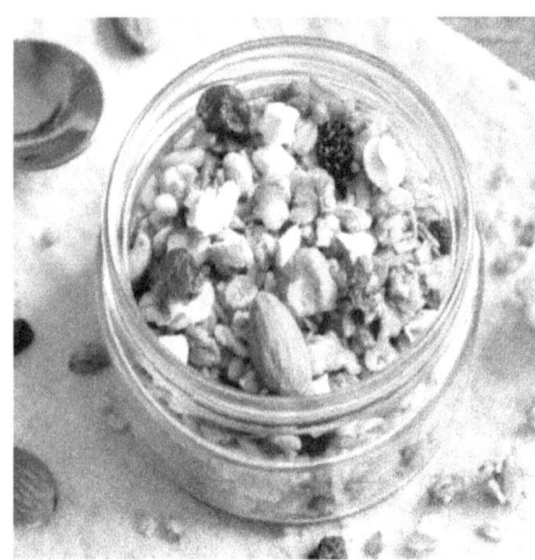

Serves:	7
Time:	1 Hour 30 Minutes
Calories:	239
Protein:	6 Grams
Fat:	11 Grams
Carbs:	32 Grams

INGREDIENTS:

- ½ Cup Maple Syrup, Pure
- ¼ Cup Coconut Oil
- ¾ Cup Coconut, Unsweetened & Shredded
- 1 Cup Almonds, Slivered
- ¾ Teaspoon Sea Salt, Fine
- 5 Cups Rolled Oats

DIRECTIONS:

1. Start by heating your oven to 250, and then mix all of your ingredients together in a bowl.

2. Spread your granola out over two baking sheets, making sure it's spread out evenly.

3. Bake for an hour and fifteen minutes, but you'll need to stir every twenty minutes.

4. Allow it to cool before serving.

Interesting Facts: Coconut oil is full of healthy fats that are absorbed easily in the human body. It is a go-to when it comes to Vegan cooking since it is a great substitute for butter and vegetable oils. It can also be used topically, in treating hair and skin. Bonus: Contains fatty acids that aid in weight loss. Double Bonus: Strengthens the immune system.

FRUITY OATMEAL

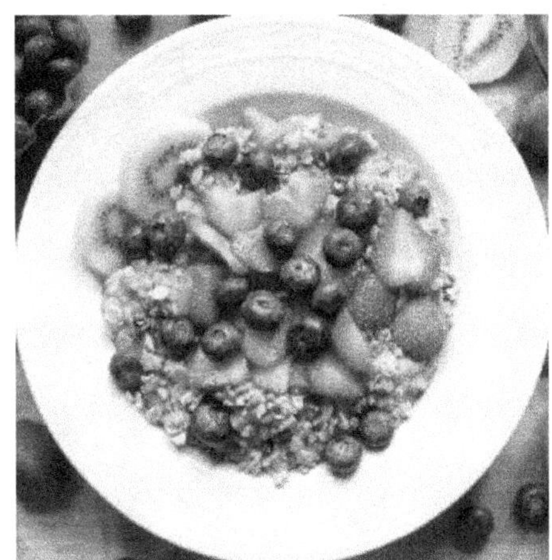

Serves: 2
Time: 25 Minutes

Calories: 230
Protein: 4.6 Grams
Fat: 5.6 Grams
Carbs: 43.8 Grams

INGREDIENTS:

- ½ Cup Apple Juice, Fresh & Frozen
- ½ Cup Oatmeal
- ½ Cup Water
- 3 Prunes, Diced
- 1 Apple, Small & Diced
- 4 Pecans, Diced
- 3 Apricots, Dehydrated, Dried & Diced
- ¼ Teaspoon Cinnamon

DIRECTIONS:

1. Start by getting out a small saucepan and mix together your apple juice and water, bringing the mixture to a boil.

2. Add a half a cup of oatmeal, cooking for a minute. Add in your pecans, cinnamon and fruit pieces. Make sure to stir. Add in your fruit when your oatmeal is nearly cool.

Interesting Facts: This spice is an absolute powerhouse and is considered one of the healthiest, beneficial spices on the plant. It's widely known for its medicinal properties. This spice is loaded with powerful antioxidants and is popular for its anti-inflammatory properties. It can reduce heart disease and lower blood sugar levels.

PLANT-BASED DIET

Chapter 8:

Lunch Recipes

PARSLEY SALAD

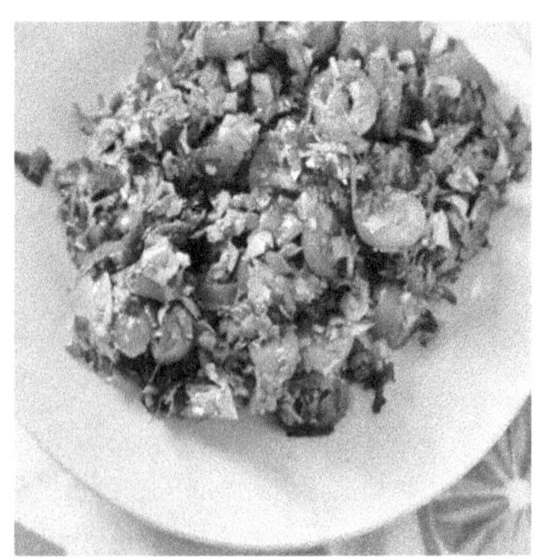

Serves: 8
Time: 30 Minutes

Calories: 165.2
Protein: 3.8 Grams
Fat: 9.1 Grams
Carbs: 20.1 Grams

INGREDIENTS:

- 3 Lemons, Juiced
- 150 Grams Flat Lea Parsley, Chopped Fine
- 1 Cup Boiled Water
- 5 Tablespoons Olive Oil

- Sea Salt & Black Pepper to Taste
- 6 Green Onions, Chopped Fine
- 1 Cup Bulgur
- 4 Tomatoes, Chopped Fine

DIRECTIONS:

1. Add your Bulgur to your water, and mix well. Put a towel on top of it to steam it. Keep it to the side, and then chop your spring onions, tomatoes and parsley. Put them in your salad bowl.

2. Pour your juice into the mixture, and then add in your olive oil, salt and pepper.

3. Put this mixture over your bulgur to serve.

Interesting Facts: This oil is a main source of dietary fat in a variety of diets. It contains many vitamins and minerals that play a part in reducing the risk of stroke and lowers cholesterol and high blood pressure and can also aid in weight loss. It is best consumed cold, as when it is heated it can lose some of its nutritive properties (although it is still great to cook with – extra virgin is best), many recommend taking a shot of cold oil olive daily! **Bonus: if you don't like the taste or texture add a shot to your smoothie.**

WATERCRESS & BLOOD ORANGE SALAD

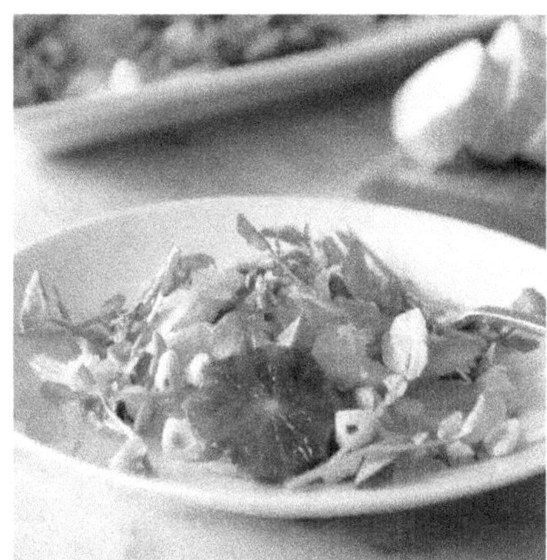

Serves: 4
Time: 10 Minutes

Calories: 94
Protein: 2 Grams
Fat: 5 Grams
Carbs: 13 Grams

INGREDIENTS:

- 1 Tablespoon Hazelnuts, Toasted & Chopped
- 2 Blood Oranges (or Navel Oranges)
- 3 Cups watercress, Stems Removed
- 1/8 Teaspoon Sea Salt, Fine
- 1 Tablespoon Lemon Juice, Fresh
- 1 Tablespoon Honey, Raw
- 1 Tablespoon Water
- 2 Tablespoons Chives, Fresh

DIRECTIONS:

1. Whisk your oil, honey, lemon juice, chives, salt and water together. Add in your watercress, tossing until it's coated.

2. Arrange the mixture onto salad plates, and top with orange slices. Drizzle with remaining liquid, and sprinkle with hazelnuts.

Interesting Facts: Lemons are popularly known as harboring loads of Vitamin C, but are also excellent sources of folate, fiber, and antioxidants. **Bonus: Helps lower cholesterol. Double Bonus: Reduces risk of cancer and high blood pressure.**

AVOCADO & RADISH SALAD

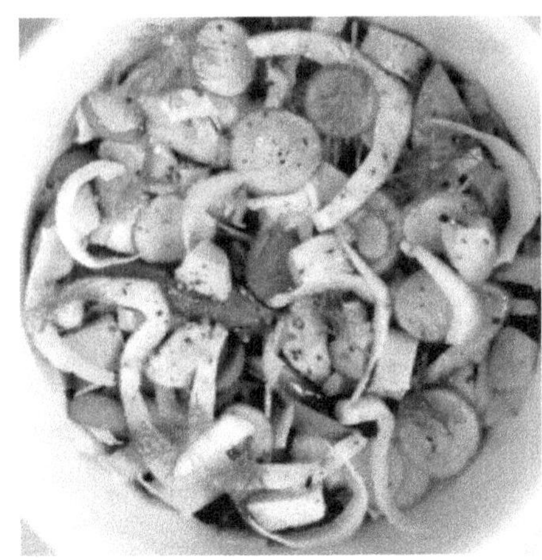

Serves: 2
Time: 10 Minutes

Calories: 223
Protein: 3 Grams
Fat: 19 Grams
Carbs: 10 Grams

INGREDIENTS:

- 1 Avocado, Sliced
- 6 Radishes, Sliced
- 2 Tomatoes, Sliced
- 1 Lettuce Head, Leaves Separated
- ½ Red Onion, Peeled & Sliced

DRESSING:

- ½ Cup Olive Oil
- ¼ Cup Lime Juice, Fresh
- ¼ Cup Apple Cider Vinegar
- 3 Cloves Garlic, Chopped Fine
- Sea Salt & Black Pepper to Taste

DIRECTIONS:

1. Spread your lettuce leaves on a platter, and then layer with your onion, tomatoes, avocado and radishes.

2. Whisk your dressing ingredients together before drizzling it over your salad.

Interesting Facts: Avocados themselves are ranked within the top five of the healthiest foods on the planet, so you know that the oil that is produced from them is too. It is loaded with healthy fats and essential fatty acids. Like race bran oil it is perfect to cook with as well! Bonus: Helps in the prevention of diabetes and lowers cholesterol levels.

ZUCCHINI & LEMON SALAD

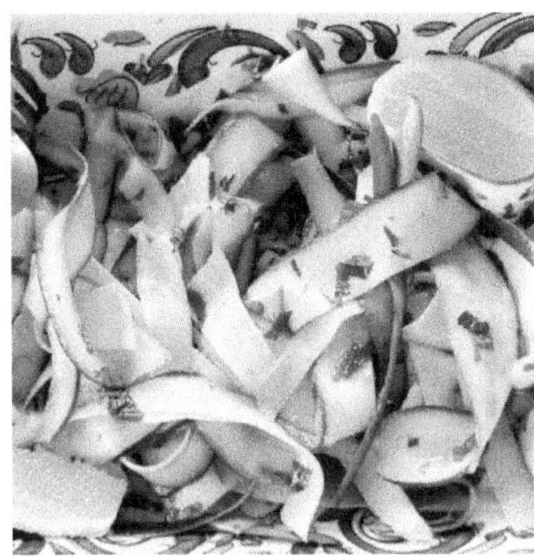

Serves: 2
Time: 3 Hours 10 Minutes

Calories: 159
Protein: 3 Grams
Fat: 14 Grams
Carbs: 7 Grams

INGREDIENTS:

- 1 Green Zucchini, Sliced into Rounds
- 1 Yellow Squash, Zucchini, Sliced into Rounds
- 1 Clove Garlic, Peeled & Chopped
- 2 Tablespoons Olive Oil
- 2 Tablespoons Basil, Fresh
- 1 Lemon, Juiced & Zested
- ¼ Cup Coconut Milk
- Sea Salt & Black Pepper to Taste

DIRECTIONS:

1. Refrigerate all ingredients for three hours before serving.

Interesting Facts: Lemons are popularly known as harboring loads of Vitamin C, but are also excellent sources of folate, fiber, and antioxidants. Bonus: Helps lower cholesterol. Double Bonus: Reduces risk of cancer and high blood pressure.

LENTIL POTATO SALAD

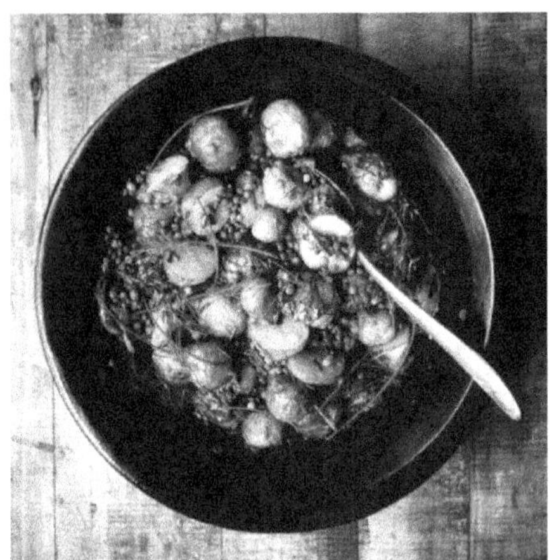

Serves: 2
Time: 35 Minutes

Calories: 400
Protein: 7 Grams
Fat: 26 Grams
Carbs: 39 Grams

INGREDIENTS:

- ½ Cup Beluga Lentils
- 8 Fingerling Potatoes
- 1 Cup Scallions, Sliced Thin
- ¼ Cup Cherry Tomatoes, Halved
- ¼ Cup Lemon Vinaigrette
- Sea Salt & Black Pepper to Taste

DIRECTIONS:

1. Bring two cups of water to simmer in a pot, adding your lentils. Cook for twenty to twenty-five minutes, and then drain. Your lentils should be tender.

2. Reduce to a simmer, cooking for fifteen minutes, and then drain. Halve your potatoes once they're cool enough to touch.

3. Put your lentils on a serving plate, and then top with scallions, potatoes and tomatoes. Drizzle with your vinaigrette, and season with salt and pepper.

Interesting Facts: Lemons are popularly known as harboring loads of Vitamin C, but are also excellent sources of folate, fiber, and antioxidants. Bonus: Helps lower cholesterol. Double Bonus: Reduces risk of cancer and high blood pressure.

OLIVE & FENNEL SALAD

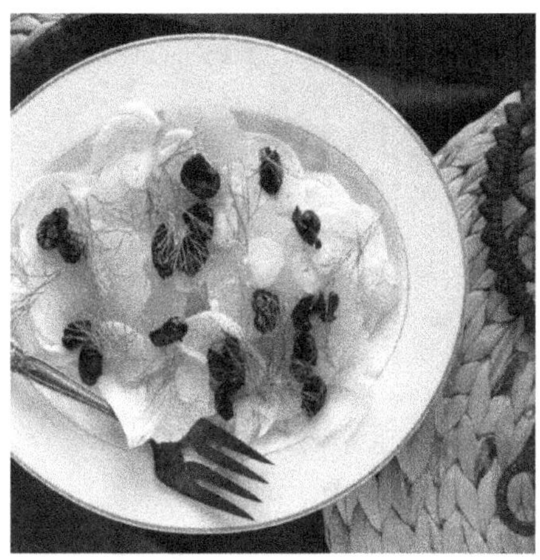

Serves:	3
Time:	5 Minutes

Calories:	331
Protein:	3 Grams
Fat:	29 Grams
Carbs:	15 Grams

INGREDIENTS:

- 6 Tablespoons Olive Oil
- 3 Fennel Bulbs, Trimmed, Cored & Quartered
- 2 Tablespoons Parsley, Fresh & Chopped
- 1 Lemon, Juiced & Zested
- 12 Black Olives
- Sea Salt & Black Pepper to Taste

DIRECTIONS:

1. Grease your baking dish, and then place your fennel in it. Make sure the cut side is up.

2. Mix your lemon zest, lemon juice, salt, pepper and oil, pouring it over your fennel.

3. Sprinkle your olives over it, and bake at 400.

4. Serve with parsley.

Interesting Facts: This oil is a main source of dietary fat in a variety of diets. It contains many vitamins and minerals that play a part in reducing the risk of stroke and lowers cholesterol and high blood pressure and can also aid in weight loss. It is best consumed cold, as when it is heated it can lose some of its nutritive properties (although it is still great to cook with – extra virgin is best), many recommend taking a shot of cold oil olive daily! Bonus: if you don't like the taste or texture add a shot to your smoothie.

BAKED OKRA & TOMATO

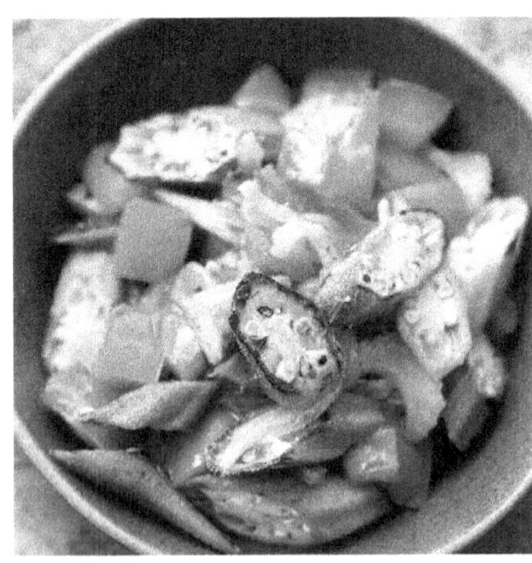

Serves:	6
Time:	1 Hour 15 Minutes
Calories:	55
Protein:	3 Grams
Fat:	0 Grams
Carbs:	12 Grams

INGREDIENTS:

- ½ cup Lime Beans, Frozen
- 4 Tomatoes, Chopped
- 8 Ounces Okra, Fresh, Washed & Stemmed, Sliced into ½ Inch Thick Slices
- 1 Onion, Sliced into Rings
- ½ Sweet Pepper, Seeded & Sliced Thin
- Pinch Crushed Red Pepper
- Sea Salt to taste

DIRECTIONS:

1. Start by heating the oven to 350, and then cook your lime beans. Drain them, and then get out a two-quarter casserole.

2. Combine everything together, and bake covered with foil for fort-five minutes.

3. Stir, and then uncover. Bake for another thirty minutes, and stir before serving.

Interesting Facts: These beans are another great multi-use veggie. They are packed with Vitamin B6, potassium, folate, and fiber. Every serving has 7.6 grams of protein. They can easily be used to make yummy veggie burgers, vegan brownies or a killer vegan Mexican meal!

RED PEPPER & BROCCOLI SALAD

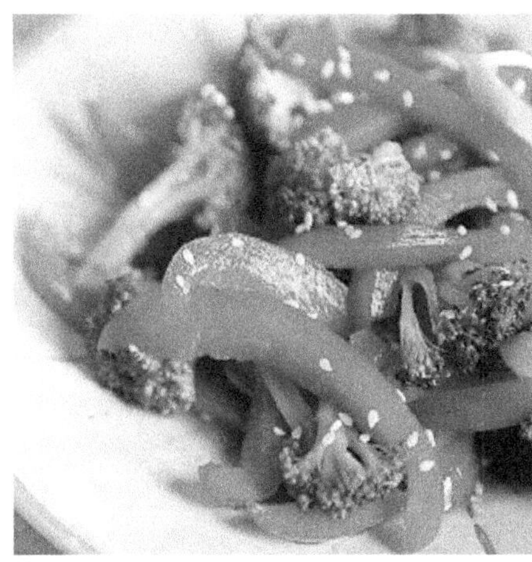

Serves:	2
Time:	15 Minutes
Calories:	185
Protein:	4 Grams
Fat:	14 Grams
Carbs:	8 Grams

INGREDIENTS:

- Ounces Lettuce Salad Mix
- 1 Head Broccoli, Chopped into Florets
- 1 Red Pepper, Seeded & Chopped

DRESSING:

- 3 Tablespoons White Wine Vinegar
- 1 Teaspoon Dijon Mustard
- 1 Clove Garlic, Peeled & Chopped Fine
- ½ Teaspoon Black Pepper
- ½ Teaspoon Sea Salt, Fine
- 2 Tablespoons Olive Oil
- 1 Tablespoon Parsley, Chopped

DIRECTIONS:

1. In boiling water, drain the broccoli it on a paper towel.

2. Whisk together all dressing ingredients.

3. Toss ingredients together before serving.

Interesting Facts: This oil is a main source of dietary fat in a variety of diets. It contains many vitamins and minerals that play a part in reducing the risk of stroke and lowers cholesterol and high blood pressure and can also aid in weight loss. It is best consumed cold, as when it is heated it can lose some of its nutritive properties (although it is still great to cook with – extra virgin is best), many recommend taking a shot of cold oil olive daily! Bonus: if you don't like the taste or texture add a shot to your smoothie.

MEDITERRANEAN WRAP

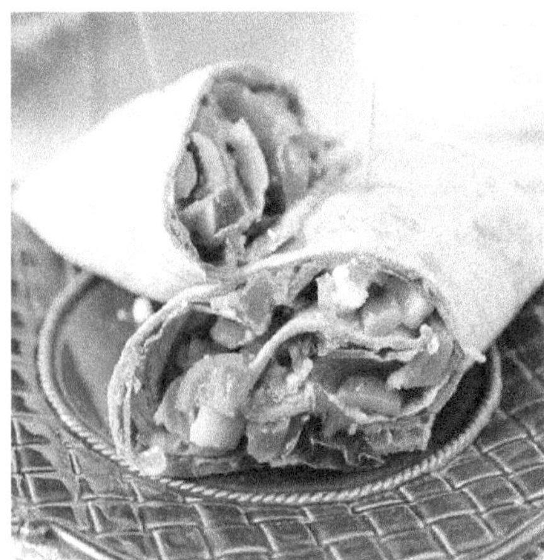

Serves: 1
Time: 10 Minutes

Calories: 428
Protein: 13 Grams
Fat: 23 Grams
Carbs: 47 Grams

INGREDIENTS:

- ¼ Cup Crispy Chickpeas
- ¼ Cup Cherry Tomatoes, Halved
- Handful Baby Spinach
- 2 Romaine Lettuce Leaves for Wrapping

- 2 Tablespoons Lemon Juice, Fresh
- ¼ Cup Hummus
- 2 Tablespoons Kalamata Olives, Quartered

DIRECTIONS:

1. Mix everything but your lettuce leaves and hummus together.

2. Put your hummus on your lettuce leaves, topping with your chickpea mixture, and then serve immediately.

Interesting Facts: Chickpeas are highly versatile and can easily be utilized in a vast array of dishes. They are infamous for making delicious hummus! They are loaded with 6 grams of protein per serving, and they are easy. You can also use chickpea water as an egg replacement known as aquafaba!

CAULIFLOWER & APPLE SALAD

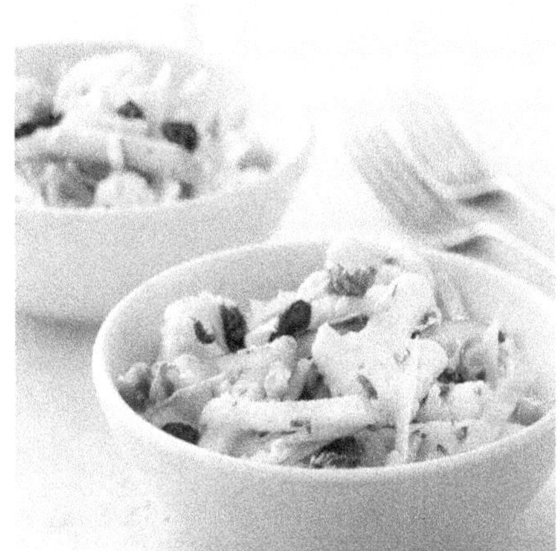

Serves: 4
Time: 25 Minutes

Calories: 198
Protein: 7 Grams
Fat: 8 Grams
Carbs: 32 Grams

INGREDIENTS:

- 3 Cups Cauliflower, Chopped into Florets
- 2 Cups Baby Kale
- 1 Sweet Apple, Cored & Chopped
- ¼ Cup Basil, Fresh & Chopped
- ¼ Cup Mint, Fresh & Chopped
- ¼ Cup Parsley, Fresh & Chopped

- 1/3 Cup Scallions, Sliced Thin
- 2 Tablespoons Yellow Raisins
- 1 Tablespoon Sun Dried Tomatoes, Chopped
- ½ Cup Miso Dressing, Optional
- ¼ Cup Roasted Pumpkin Seeds, Optional

DIRECTIONS:

1. Combine everything together, tossing before serving.

Interesting Facts: This vegetable is an extremely high source of vitamin A, vitamin B1, B2 and B3.

MAC & "CHEESE"

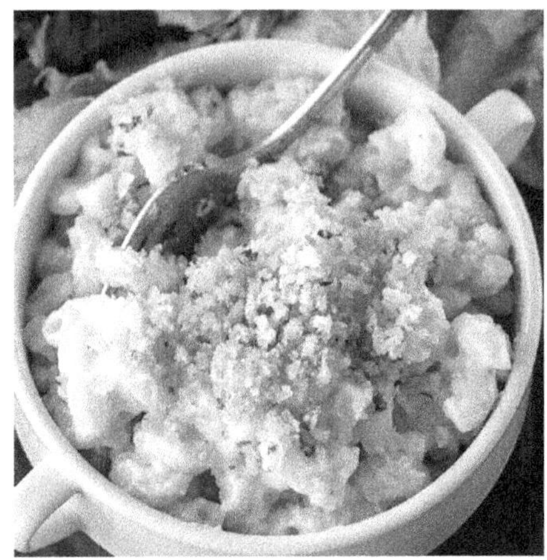

Serves: 6
Time: 40 Minutes

Calories: 848
Protein: 70 Grams
Fat: 8.4 Grams
Carbs: 140.1 Grams

INGREDIENTS:

- Milk Substitute
- 16 Ounces Elbow Macaroni, Whole Wheat
- 16 Ounces Vegan Mayonnaise
- 3 Cups Nutritional Yeast
- Whole Wheat Bread Crumbs
- Sea Salt & Black Pepper to Taste

DIRECTIONS:

1. Make your noodles as the package instructs. Drain them, and then add in your ingredients, and mix well.

2. Add in your milk substitute, stirring until creamy.

3. Pour your ingredients into a baking dish and then sprinkle your bread crumbs on top.

4. Bake until it's golden brown, which will take about a half hour.

Interesting Facts: A classic staple, whole wheat is incredibly beneficial to your health. Be sure to steer clear of multigrain, however, and go for the stuff marked 100% whole grain to make sure you are getting exactly what you need!

SUMMER CHICKPEA SALAD

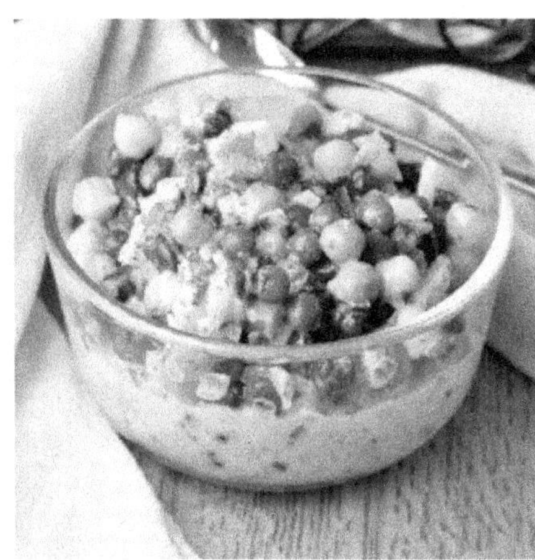

Serves: 4
Time: 15 Minutes

Calories: 145
Protein: 4 Grams
Fat: 7.5 Grams
Carbs: 16 Grams

INGREDIENTS:

- 1 ½ Cups Cherry Tomatoes, Halved
- 1 Cup English Cucumber, Slices
- 1 Cup Chickpeas, Canned, Unsalted, Drained & Rinsed
- ¼ Cup Red Onion, Slivered
- 2 Tablespoon Olive Oil
- 1 ½ Tablespoons Lemon Juice, Fresh
- 1 ½ Tablespoons Lemon Juice, Fresh
- Sea Salt & Black Pepper to Taste

DIRECTIONS:

1. Mix everything together, and toss to combine before serving.

Interesting Facts: Chickpeas are highly versatile and can easily be utilized in a vast array of dishes. They are infamous for making delicious hummus! They are loaded with 6 grams of protein per serving, and they are easy. You can also use chickpea water as an egg replacement known as aquafaba!

EDAMAME SALAD

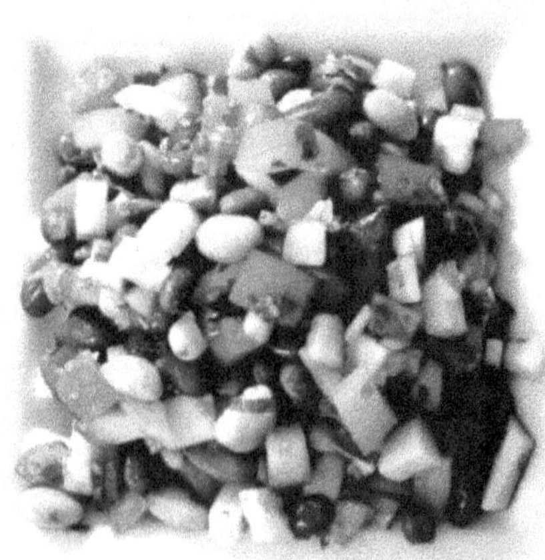

Serves: 1
Time: 15 Minutes

Calories: 299
Protein: 20 Grams
Fat: 9 Grams
Carbs: 38 Grams

INGREDIENTS:

- ¼ Cup Red Onion, Chopped
- 1 Cup Corn Kernels, Fresh
- 1 Cup Edamame Beans, Shelled & Thawed
- 1 Red Bell Pepper, Chopped
- 2-3 Tablespoons Lime Juice, Fresh
- 5-6 Basil Leaves, Fresh & Sliced
- 5-6 Mint Leaves, Fresh & Sliced
- Sea Salt & Black Pepper to Taste

DIRECTIONS:

1. Place everything into a Mason jar, and then seal the jar tightly. Shake well before serving.

Interesting Facts: Whole corn is a fantastic source of phosphorus, magnesium, and B vitamins. It also promotes healthy digestion and contains heart-healthy antioxidants. It is important to seek out organic corn in order to bypass all of the genetically modified product that is out on the market.

CORN & BLACK BEAN SALAD

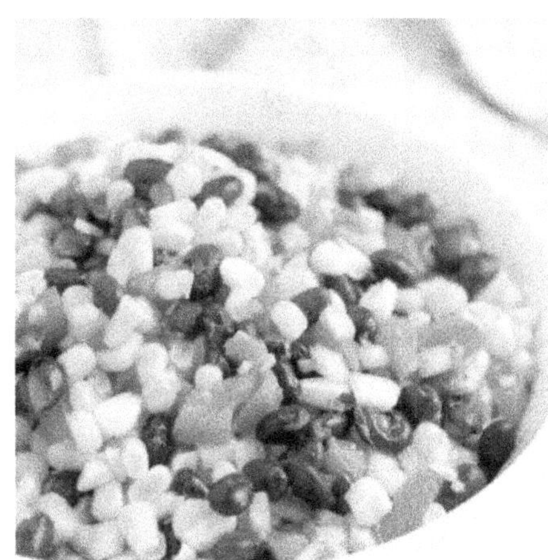

Serves:	6
Time:	10 Minutes
Calories:	159
Protein:	6.4 Grams
Fat:	5.6 Grams
Carbs:	23.7 Grams

INGREDIENTS:

- ¼ Cup Cilantro, Fresh & Chopped
- 1 Can Corn, Drained (10 Ounces)
- 1/8 Cup Red Onion, Chopped
- 1 Can Black Beans, Drained (15 Ounces)
- 1 Tomato, Chopped
- 3 Tablespoons Lemon Juice, Fresh
- 2 Tablespoons Olive Oil
- Sea Salt & Black Pepper to Taste

DIRECTIONS:

1. Mix everything together, and then refrigerates until cool. Serve cold.

Interesting Facts: Whole corn is a fantastic source of phosphorus, magnesium, and B vitamins. It also promotes healthy digestion and contains heart-healthy antioxidants. It is important to seek out organic corn in order to bypass all of the genetically modified product that is out on the market.

BUTTER BEAN HUMMUS

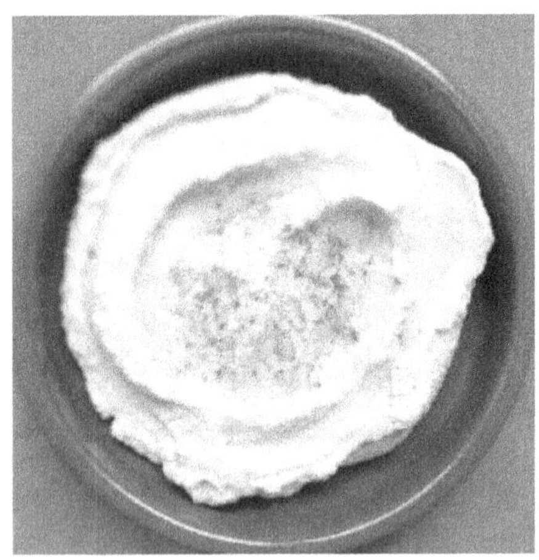

Serves: 4
Time: 5 Minutes

Calories: 150
Protein: 8 Grams
Fat: 4 Grams
Carbs: 23 Grams

INGREDIENTS:

- 1 Can Butter Beans, Drained & Rinsed
- 4 Sprigs Parsley, Minced
- 1 Tablespoon Olive Oil
- ½ Lemon, Juiced
- 2 Cloves Garlic, Minced
- Sea Salt to Taste

DIRECTIONS:

1. Blend and serve as a dip with fresh vegetables.

Interesting Facts: This oil is a main source of dietary fat in a variety of diets. It contains many vitamins and minerals that play a part in reducing the risk of stroke and lowers cholesterol and high blood pressure and can also aid in weight loss. It is best consumed cold, as when it is heated it can lose some of its nutritive properties (although it is still great to cook with – extra virgin is best), many recommend taking a shot of cold oil olive daily! Bonus: if you don't like the taste or texture add a shot to your smoothie.

SPINACH & ORANGE SALAD

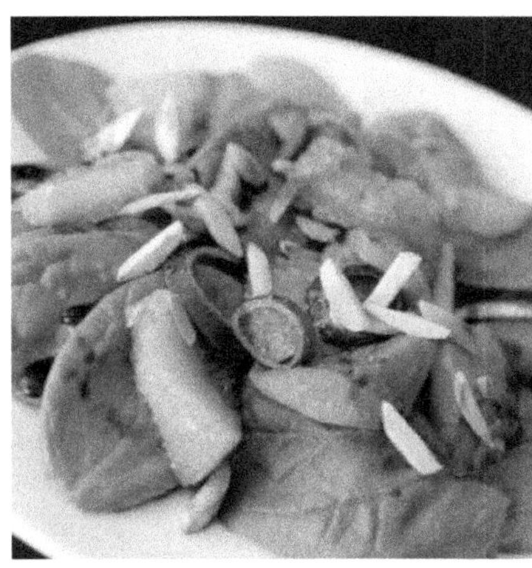

Serves:	6
Time:	15 Minutes
Calories:	99
Protein:	2.5 Grams
Fat:	5 Grams
Carbs:	13.1 Grams

INGREDIENTS:

- ¼ -1/3 Cup Vegan Dressing

- 3 Oranges, Medium, Peeled, Seeded & Sectioned

- ¾ lb. Spinach, Fresh & Torn

- 1 Red Onion, Medium, Sliced & Separated into Rings

DIRECTIONS:

1. Toss everything together, and serve with dressing.

Interesting Facts: Spinach is one of the most superb green veggies out there. Each serving is packed with 3 grams of protein and is a highly encouraged component of the plant-based diet.

FRUITY KALE SALAD

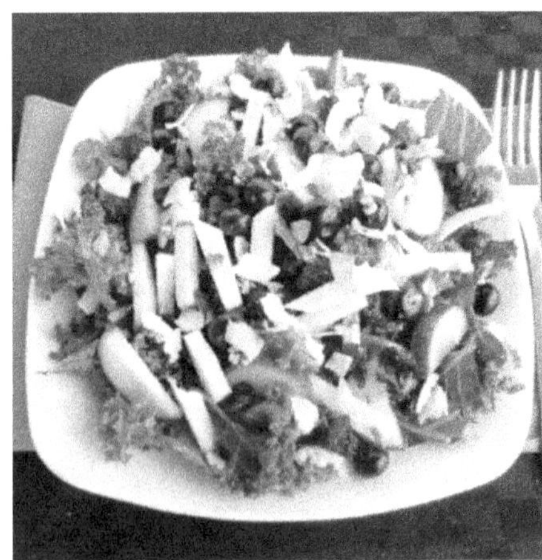

Serves: 4
Time: 30 Minutes

Calories: 220
Protein: 4 Grams
Fat: 17 Grams
Carbs: 16 Grams

INGREDIENTS:

Salad:

- 10 Ounces Baby Kale
- ½ Cup Pomegranate Arils
- 1 Tablespoon Olive Oil
- 1 Apple, Sliced

Dressing:

- 3 Tablespoons Apple Cider Vinegar
- 3 Tablespoons Olive Oil
- 1 Tablespoon Tahini Sauce (Optional)
- Sea Salt & Black Pepper to Taste

DIRECTIONS:

1. Wash and dry the kale. If kale is too expensive, you can also use lettuce, arugula or spinach. Take the stems out, and chop it.

2. Combine all of your salad ingredients together.

3. Combine all of your dressing ingredients together before drizzling it over the salad to serve.

Interesting Facts: Kale is the latest superfood of the Vegan world. It is a favorite when deciding to eliminate meat from your diet as it is very high in iron, vitamin K and potassium. It is also extremely high in fibre and vitamin A.

Chapter 9:

Soups and Stews

BLACK EYED PEAS STEW

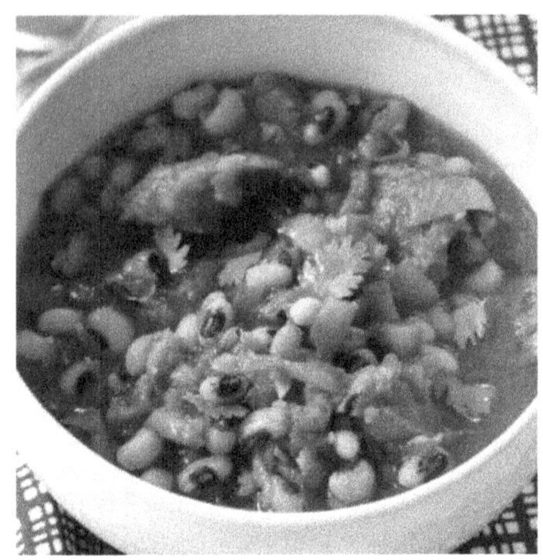

Serves: 5
Time: 30 Minutes

Calories: 338
Protein: 21 Grams
Fat: 4 Grams
Carbs: 58 Grams

INGREDIENTS:

- 1 Can Tomatoes, Crushed

- ¼ Teaspoon Cayenne

- 1 Clove Garlic

- 2 Tablespoons Olive Oil

- 1 Onion

- 2 Cans Black Eyed Peas, Drained

- 8 Ounces Okra, Frozen & Thawed

- Sea Salt to Taste

DIRECTIONS:

1. Start by brown your onion using olive oil, and then add in your garlic and cayenne. Cook for another minute.

2. Mix in all of your remaining ingredients, simmering until your okra becomes soft.

Interesting Facts: Black Eyed peas are infamous for making delicious hummus! They are loaded with 6 grams of protein per serving, and they are easy. You can also use chickpea water as an egg replacement known as aquafaba!

RED LENTIL SOUP

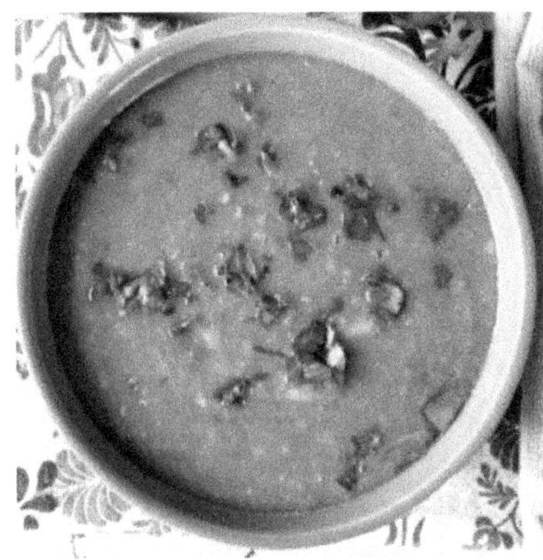

Serves: 4
Time: 50 Minutes

Calories: 188
Protein: 12.5 Grams
Fat: 1.2 Grams
Carbs: 33.6 Grams

INGREDIENTS:

- 1 Teaspoon Paprika
- 4 Cups Vegetable Stock
- ¼ Cup Onion, Chopped Fine
- 1 Cup Lentil, Red, Washed & Cleaned
- ½ Cup Potato, Peeled & Diced
- Sea Salt & Black Pepper to Taste

DIRECTIONS:

1. Rinse your lentils under cold water, and then get out a medium pot.

2. Place your red lentils, potatoes, stock, onion and paprika in the pot.

3. Allow it to simmer.

4. Put the lid on loosely, and cook until your lentils are tender. This will take roughly thirty minutes.

5. Add your salt and pepper, put a cup of the soup in the food processor, and then place the blended soup back into the pot.

6. Serve warm.

Interesting Facts: Potatoes are a great starchy source of potassium and protein. They are pretty inexpensive if you are one that is watching their budget. Bonus: Very heart healthy

QUINOA WITH NECTARINE SLAW

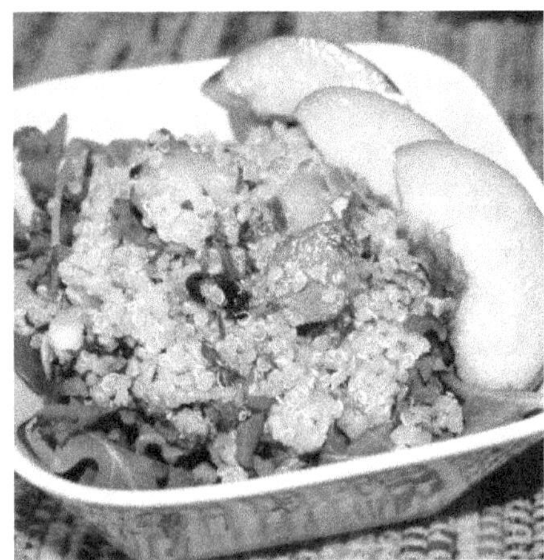

Serves: 2
Time: 20 Minutes

Calories: 396
Protein: 11 Grams
Fat: 18 Grams
Carbs: 52 Grams

INGREDIENTS:

- ½ Cup Kale, Chopped
- 1/3 Cup Pumpkin Seeds, Roasted
- 3 Tablespoons Lemon Vinaigrette
- 1 Teaspoon Nutritional Yeast (Optional)

- 1/3 Cup Scallions, Sliced Thin
- 1 Cup Quinoa, Cooked & Room Temperature
- 2 Nectarines, Chopped into ½ Inch Wedges
- ½ Cup White Cabbage, Shredded

DIRECTIONS:

1. Combine everything together in a bowl before serving.

Interesting Facts: Pumpkin seeds are popularly known as a yummy snack, and can also be easily incorporated into soups, yogurt, salads, and more! They are loaded with iron, Vitamins C, E, and K, and essential omega-3s.

THAI SQUASH SOUP

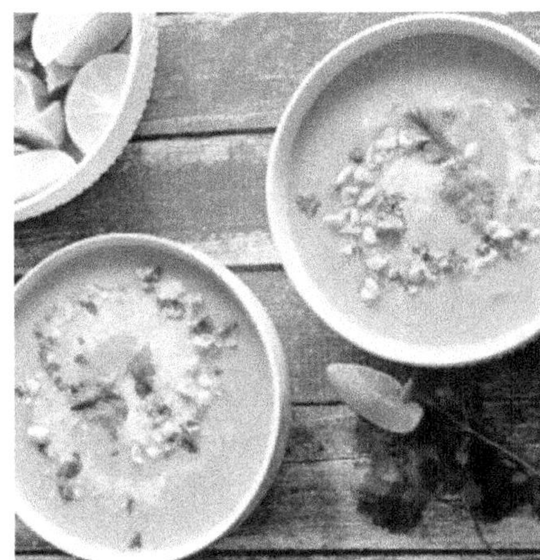

Serves: 2
Time: 30 Minutes

Calories: 717.3
Protein: 10.3 Grams
Fat: 48.3 Grams
Carbs: 77.4 Grams

INGREDIENTES:

- 1 Teaspoon Curry Powder
- 1 Tablespoon Olive Oil
- 1 Red Onion, Chopped
- 1 Pint Vegetable Stock
- 1 Butter Squash, Chunked
- 1 Can Coconut Milk (Roughly 13.5 Ounces)

DIRECTIONS:

1. Get out a pan and heat your olive oil. Once it's heated, add in your onion and cook to soften. This should take two to three minutes. Add your butternut squash, stock to taste, and curry powder.

2. Simmer. The squash should become tender.

3. Stir in your coconut milk, and then blend until smooth.

4. Return it to the pan to warm, and season with salt and pepper before serving.

Interesting Facts: Coconut oil is full of healthy fats that are absorbed easily in the human body. It is a go-to when it comes to Vegan cooking since it is a great substitute for butter and vegetable oils. It can also be used topically, in treating hair and skin. Bonus: Contains fatty acids that aid in weight loss. Double Bonus: Strengthens the immune system.

WHITE BEAN & SPINACH SOUP

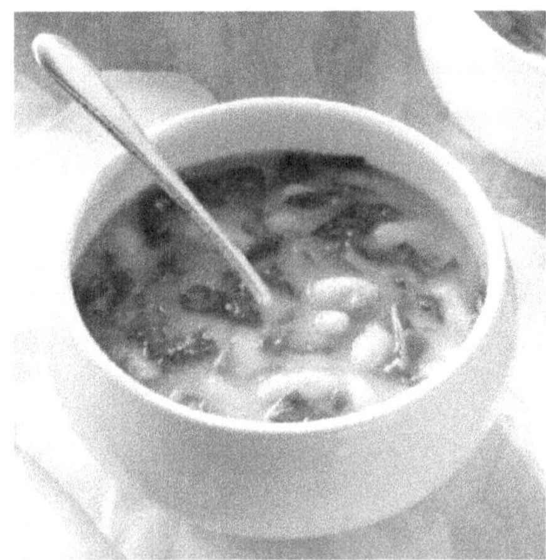

Serves:	4
Time:	25 Minutes
Calories:	218
Protein:	12 Grams
Fat:	3.3 Grams
Carbs:	37.9 Grams

INGREDIENTS:

- 3 Cups Baby Spinach, Cleaned & Trimmed
- 1 Can White Beans (Roughly 14.5 Ounces)
- 3-4 Cups Vegetable Stock, Homemade
- 1 Shallot, Diced Fine
- 1 Clove Garlic, Minced Fine
- 14.5 Ounces Tomatoes, Diced
- 1 Teaspoon Rosemary
- ½ Cup Shell Pasta, Whole Wheat
- 2 Teaspoons Olive Oil
- Red Pepper Flakes to Taste
- Black Pepper to Taste

DIRECTIONS:

1. Heat olive oil in a saucepan before sautéing your garlic and shallots

2. Add in your rosemary, beans, broth and tomatoes. Season with your red pepper flakes and black pepper.

3. Put your pasta in, cooking for ten minutes, and then add in your spinach. Cook until it's wilted.

Interesting Facts: Spinach is one of the most superb green veggies out there. Each serving is packed with 3 grams of protein and is a highly encouraged component of the plant-based diet.

CABBAGE & BEET STEW

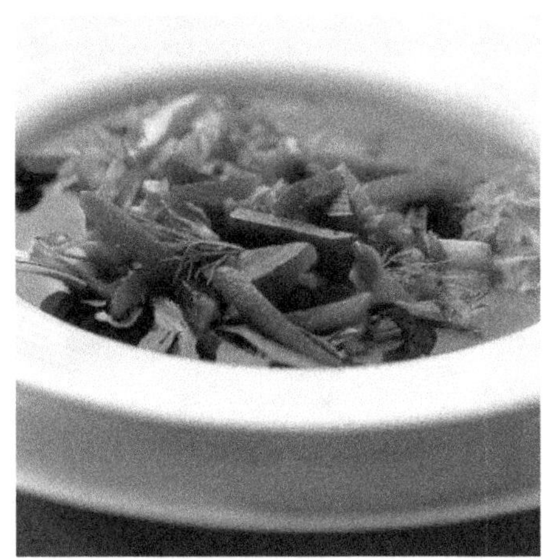

Serves: 4
Time: 30 Minutes

Calories: 95
Protein: 1 Gram
Fat: 7 Grams
Carbs: 10 Grams

INGREDIENTS:

- 2 Tablespoons Olive Oil
- 3 Cups Vegetable Broth
- 2 Tablespoons Lemon Juice, Fresh
- ½ Teaspoon Garlic Powder
- ½ Cup Carrots, Shredded

- 2 Cups Cabbage, Shredded
- 1 Cup Beets, Shredded
- Dill for Garnish
- ½ Teaspoon Onion Powder
- Sea Salt & Black Pepper to Taste

DIRECTIONS:

1. Heat oil in a pot, and then sauté your vegetables.

2. Pour your broth in, mixing in your seasoning. Simmer until it's cooked through, and then top with dill.

Interesting Facts: This oil is a main source of dietary fat in a variety of diets. It contains many vitamins and minerals that play a part in reducing the risk of stroke and lowers cholesterol and high blood pressure and can also aid in weight loss. It is best consumed cold, as when it is heated it can lose some of its nutritive properties (although it is still great to cook with – extra virgin is best), many recommend taking a shot of cold oil olive daily! Bonus: if you don't like the taste or texture add a shot to your smoothie.

Chapter 10:

Dinner Recipes

SESAME BOK CHOY

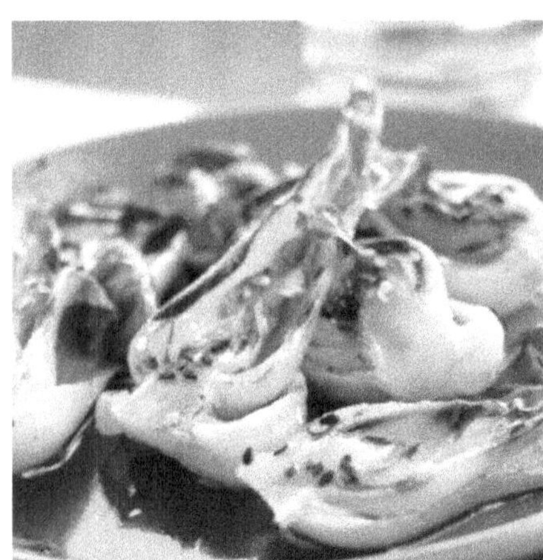

Serves: 4
Time: 13 Minutes

Calories: 76
Protein: 4.4 Grams
Fat: 2.7 Grams
Carbs: 9.8 Grams

INGREDIENTS:

- 1 Head Bok Choy
- 1 Teaspoon Canola Oil
- 1/3 Cup Green Onion, Chopped
- 1 Tablespoon Brown Sugar
- 1 ½ Tablespoon Soy Sauce, Light
- 1 Tablespoon Rice Wine
- ½ Teaspoon Ginger, Ground
- 1 Tablespoon Sesame Seeds

DIRECTIONS:

1. Cut the stems and tops of your bok choy into one inch pieces.

2. Mix together all remaining ingredients in a bowl.

3. Add your bok choy, and top with your dressing.

4. Fry until tender, which should take eight to ten minutes.

Interesting Facts: Sesame seeds can be easily added to crackers, bread, salads, and stir-fry meals. Bonus: Help in lowering cholesterol and high blood pressure. Double bonus: Help with asthma, arthritis, and migraines!

TOFU & ASPARAGUS STIR FRY

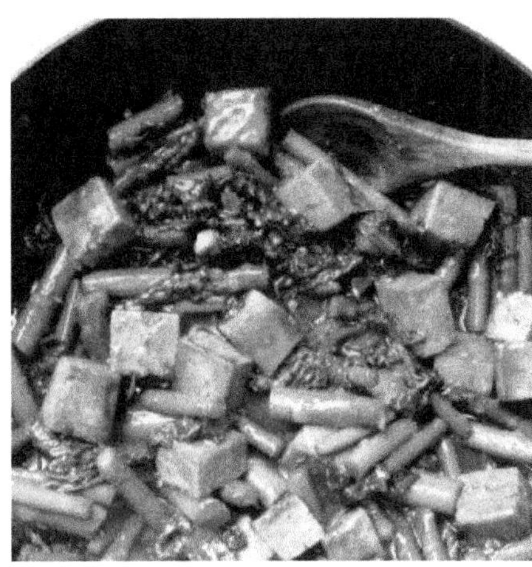

Serves:	3
Time:	20 Minutes

Calories:	380
Protein:	22 Grams
Fat:	24 Grams
Carbs:	27 Grams

INGREDIENTS:

- 1 Tablespoon Ginger, Peeled & Grated
- 8 Ounces Firm Tofu, Chopped into Slices
- 4 Green Onions, Sliced Thin
- Toasted Sesame Oil to Taste
- 1 Bunch Asparagus, Trimmed & Chopped
- 1 Handful Cashew Nuts, Chopped & Toasted
- 2 Tablespoons Hoisin Sauce
- 1 Lime, Juiced & Zested
- 1 Handful Mint, Fresh & Chopped
- 1 Handful Basil, Fresh & Chopped
- 3 Cloves Garlic, Chopped
- 3 Handfuls Spinach, Chopped
- Pinch Sea Salt

DIRECTIONS:

1. Get out a wok and heat up your oil. Add in your tofu, cooking for a few minutes.

2. Put your tofu to the side, and then sauté your red pepper flakes, ginger, salt, onions and asparagus for a minute.

3. Mix in your spinach, garlic, and cashews, cooking for another two minutes.

4. Add your tofu back in, and then drizzle in your lime juice, lime zest, hoisin sauce, cooking for another half a minute.

5. Remove it from heat, adding in your mint and basil.

Interesting Facts: Sesame seeds can be easily added to crackers, bread, salads, and stir-fry meals. Bonus: Help in lowering cholesterol and high blood pressure. Double bonus: Help with asthma, arthritis, and migraines!

TOMATO GAZPACHO

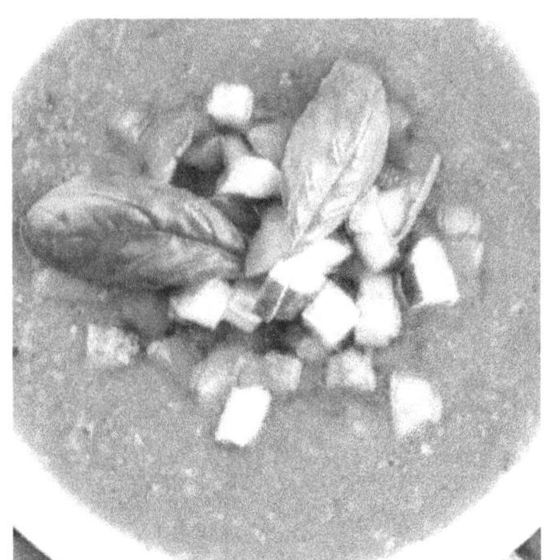

Serves: 6
Time: 2 Hours 25 Minutes

Calories: 181
Protein: 3 Grams
Fat: 14 Grams
Carbs: 14 Grams

INGREDIENTS:

- 2 Tablespoons + 1 Teaspoon Red Wine Vinegar, Divided
- ½ Teaspoon Pepper
- 1 Teaspoon Sea Salt
- 1 Avocado,
- ¼ Cup Basil, Fresh & Chopped

- 3 Tablespoons + 2 Teaspoons Olive Oil, Divided
- 1 Clove Garlic, crushed
- 1 Red Bell Pepper, Sliced & Seeded
- 1 Cucumber, Chunked
- 2 ½ lbs. Large Tomatoes, Cored & Chopped

DIRECTIONS:

1. Place half of your cucumber, bell pepper, and ¼ cup of each tomato in a bowl, covering. Set it in the fried.

2. Puree your remaining tomatoes, cucumber and bell pepper with garlic, three tablespoons oil, two tablespoons of vinegar, sea salt and black pepper into a blender, blending until smooth. Transfer it to a bowl, and chill for two hours.

3. Chop the avocado, adding it to your chopped vegetables, adding your remaining oil, vinegar, salt, pepper and basil.

4. Ladle your tomato puree mixture into bowls, and serve with chopped vegetables as a salad.

Interesting Facts: Avocados themselves are ranked within the top five of the healthiest foods on the planet, so you know that the oil that is produced from them is too. It is loaded with healthy fats and essential fatty acids. Like race bran oil it is perfect to cook with as well! Bonus: Helps in the prevention of diabetes and lowers cholesterol levels.

SIMPLE CHILI

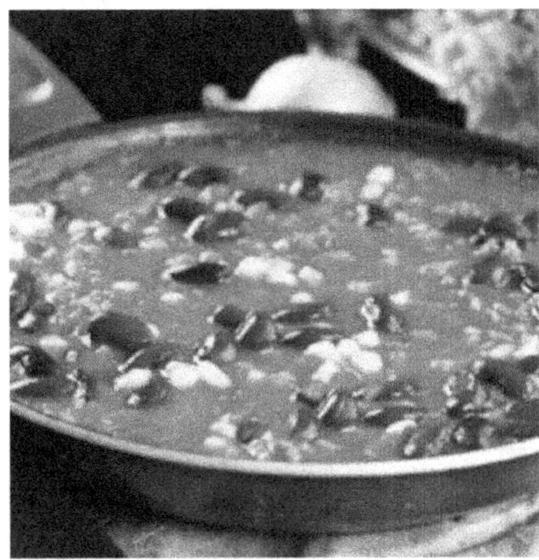

Serves:	4
Time:	30 Minutes
Calories:	160
Protein:	8 Grams
Fat:	3 Grams
Carbs:	29 Grams

INGREDIENTS:

- 1 Onion, Diced

- 1 Teaspoon Olive Oil

- 3 Cloves Garlic, Minced

- 28 Ounces Tomatoes, Canned

- ¼ Cup Tomato Paste

- 14 Ounces Kidney Beans, Canned, Rinsed & Dried

- 2-3 Teaspoons Chili Powder

- ¼ Cup Cilantro, Fresh (or Parsley)

- ¼ Teaspoon Sea Salt, Fine

DIRECTIONS:

1. Get out a pot, and sauté your onion and garlic in your oil at the bottom cook for five minutes. Add in your tomato paste, tomatoes, beans, and chili powder. Season with salt.

2. Allow it to simmer for ten to twenty minutes.

3. Garnish with cilantro or parsley to serve.

Interesting Facts: Kidney beans are packed with Vitamin B6, potassium, folate, and fiber. Every serving has 7.6 grams of protein. They can easily be used to make yummy veggie burgers, vegan brownies or a killer vegan Mexican meal!

CAULIFLOWER RICE TABBOULEH

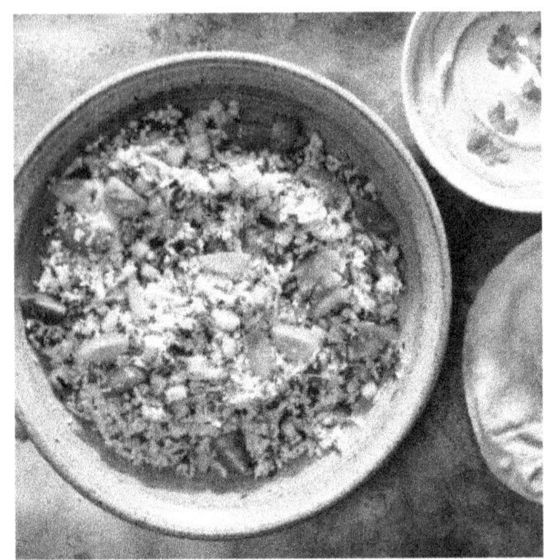

Serves: 4
Time: 20 Minutes

Calories: 220
Protein: 7 Grams
Fat: 15 Grams
Carbs: 20 Grams

INGREDIENTS:

- 4 Cups Cauliflower Rice
- 1 ½ Cups Cherry Tomatoes, Quartered
- 3-4 Tablespoons Olive Oil
- 1 Cup Parsley, Fresh & Chopped
- 1 Cup Mint, Fresh & Chopped
- 1 Cup Snap Peas, Sliced Thin
- 1 Small Cucumber, Cut into ¼ Inch Pieces
- ¼ Cup Scallions, Sliced Thin
- 3-4 Tablespoons Lemon Juice, Fresh
- 1 Teaspoon Sea Salt, Fine
- ½ Teaspoon Black Pepper

DIRECTIONS:

1. Get out a bowl and combine your cauliflower rice, tomatoes, mint, parsley, cucumbers, scallions and snap peas together. Toss until combined.

2. Add your olive oil and lemon juice before tossing again. Season with salt and pepper.

Interesting Facts: Cauliflower: This vegetable is an extremely high source of vitamin A, vitamin B1, B2 and B3.

DIJON MAPLE BURGERS

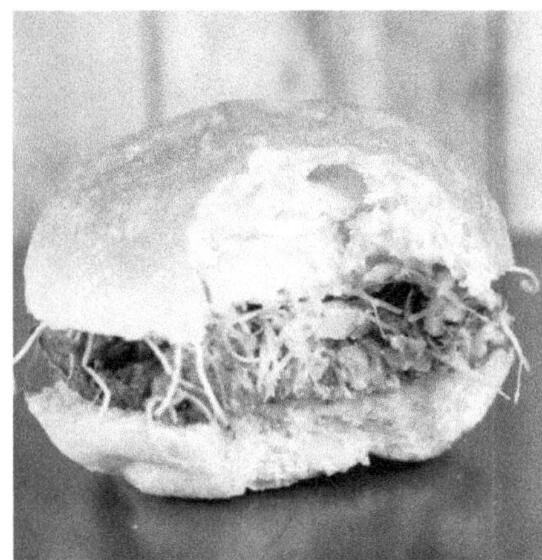

Serves: 12
Time: 50 Minutes

Calories: 200
Protein: 8 Grams
Fat: 11 Grams
Carbs: 21 Grams

INGREDIENTS:

- 1 Red Bell Pepper
- 19 Ounces Can Chickpeas, Rinsed & Drained
- 1 Cup Almonds, Ground
- 2 Teaspoons Dijon Mustard
- 1 Teaspoon Oregano
- ½ Teaspoon Sage
- 1 Cup Spinach, Fresh
- 1 – ½ Cups Rolled Oats
- 1 Clove Garlic, Pressed
- ½ Lemon, Juiced
- 2 Teaspoons Maple Syrup, Pure

DIRECTIONS:

1. Get out a baking sheet. Line it with parchment paper.

2. Cut your red pepper in half and then take the seeds out. Place it on your baking sheet, and roast in the oven while you prepare your other ingredients.

3. Process your chickpeas, almonds, mustard and maple syrup together in a food processor.

4. Add in your lemon juice, oregano, sage, garlic and spinach, processing again. Make sure it's combined, but don't puree it.

5. Once your red bell pepper is softened, which should roughly take ten minutes, add this to the processor as well. Add in your oats, mixing well.

6. Form twelve patties, cooking in the oven for a half hour. They should be browned.

Interesting Facts: Spinach is one of the most superb green veggies out there. Each serving is packed with 3 grams of protein and is a highly encouraged component of the plant-based diet.

GRILLED EGGPLANT STEAKS

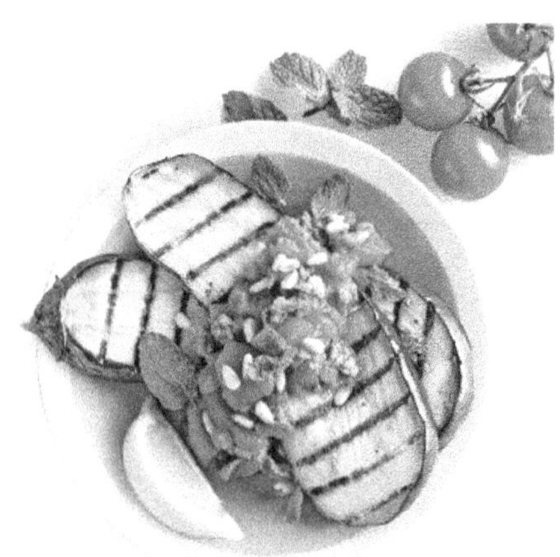

Serves:	6
Time:	35 Minutes
Calories:	86
Protein:	8 Grams
Fat:	7 Grams
Carbs:	12 Grams

INGREDIENTS:

- 4 Roma Tomatoes, Diced
- 8 Ounces Feta, Diced
- 2 Eggplants
- 1 Tablespoon Olive Oil

- 1 Cup Parsley, Chopped
- 1 Cucumber, Diced
- Sea Salt & Black Pepper to Taste

DIRECTIONS:

1. Slice your eggplants into three thick steaks, and then drizzle with oil. Season then grill for four minutes per side in a pan.

2. Top with the remaining ingredients.

Interesting Facts: Eggplant has a variety of vital vitamins and minerals within it's compound. It is high in folic acid, vitamin C, manganese and vitamin K. It aids weight lose and cognitive function. Eggplant is a great meat replacement in a lasagna!

SUSHI BOWL

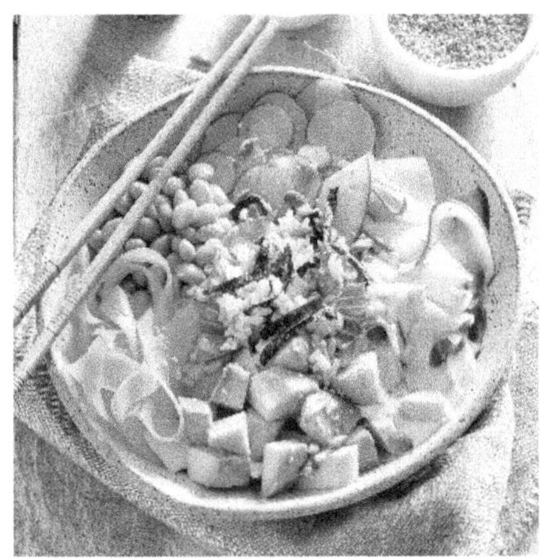

Serves: 1
Time: 40 Minutes

Calories: 467
Protein: 22 Grams
Fat: 20 Grams
Carbs: 56 Grams

INGREDIENTS:

- ½ Cup Edamame Beans, Shelled & Fresh
- ¾ Cup Brown Rice, Cooked
- ½ Cup Spinach, Chopped
- ¼ Cup Bell Pepper, Sliced
- ¼ Cup Avocado, Sliced
- ¼ Cup Cilantro, Fresh & Chopped
- 1 Scallion, Chopped
- ¼ Nori Sheet
- 1-2 Tablespoons Tamari
- 1 Tablespoon Sesame Seeds, Optional

DIRECTIONS:

1. Steam your edamame beans, and then assemble your edamame, rice, avocado, spinach, cilantro, scallions and bell pepper into a bowl.

2. Cut the nori into ribbons, sprinkling it on top, drizzling with tamari and sesame seeds before serving.

Interesting Facts: Avocados are known as miracle fruits in the world of Veganism. They are a true super-fruit and incredibly beneficial. They are one of the best things to eat if you are looking to incorporate more fatty acids in your diet. They are also loaded with 20 various minerals and vitamins. Plus, they are easy to incorporate into dishes all throughout the day!

CAULIFLOWER STEAKS

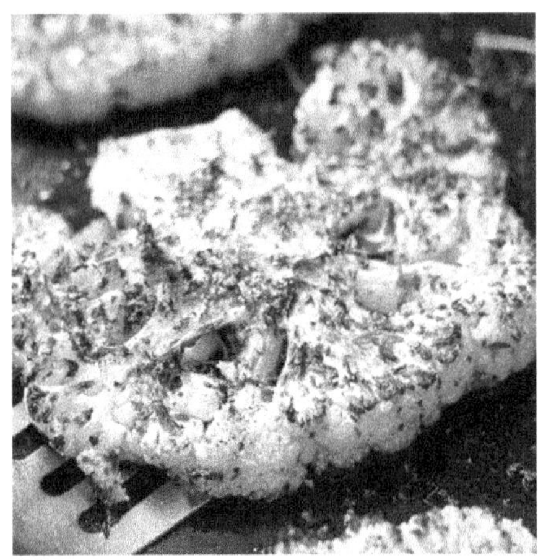

Serves: 4
Time: 30 Minutes

Calories: 167
Protein: 6 Grams
Fat: 13 Grams
Carbs: 10 Grams

INGREDIENTS:

- ¼ Teaspoon Black Pepper
- ½ Teaspoon Sea Salt, Fine
- 1 Tablespoon Olive Oil
- 1 Head Cauliflower, Large
- ¼ Cup Creamy Hummus
- 2 Tablespoons Lemon Sauce
- ½ Cup Peanuts, Crushed (Optional)

DIRECTIONS:

1. Start by heating your oven to 425.

2. Cut your cauliflower stems, and then remove the leaves. Put the cut side down, and then slice half down the middle. Cut into ¾ inch steaks. If you cut them thinner, they could fall apart.

3. Arrange them in a single layer on a baking sheet, drizzling with oil. Season and bake for twenty to twenty-five minutes. They should be lightly browned and tender.

4. Spread your hummus on the steaks, drizzling with your lemon sauce. Top with peanuts if you're using it.

Interesting Facts: Cauliflower: This vegetable is an extremely high source of vitamin A, vitamin B1, B2 and B3.

PESTO & TOMATO QUINOA

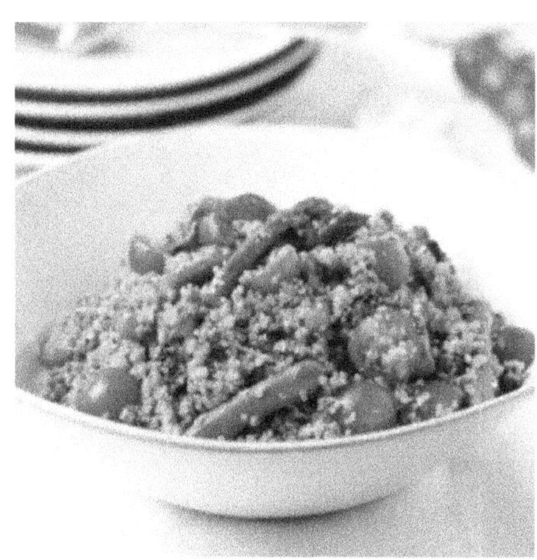

Serves: 1
Time: 25 Minutes

Calories: 535
Protein: 20 Grams
Fat: 23 Grams
Carbs: 69 Grams

INGREDIENTS:

- 1 Teaspoon Olive Oil
- 1 Cup Onion, Chopped
- 1 Cup Zucchini, Chopped
- 1 Clove Garlic, Minced
- 1 Tomato, Chopped
- Pinch Sea Salt
- 2 Tablespoons Sun Dried Tomatoes, Chopped
- 2-3 Tablespoons Basil Pesto
- 1 Cup Spinach, Chopped
- 2 Cups Quinoa, Cooked
- 1 Tablespoon Nutritional Yeast, Optional

DIRECTIONS:

1. Heat your oil in a skillet, and sauté your onion over medium-high heat. This should take five minutes, and then add in your garlic, cooking for another minute. Add in your sea salt and zucchini.

2. Cook for about five-minute and then add in your sun dried tomatoes, and mix well.

3. Toss your pesto in, and then mix well.

4. Layer your spinach, quinoa and then zucchini mixture on a plate, topping with nutritional yeast if desired.

Interesting Facts: Quinoa is an important staple for anyone looking to get the most out of a plant based diet.

RATATOUILLE

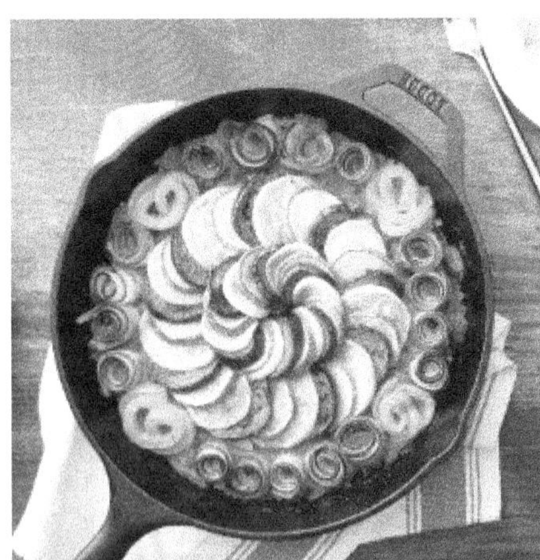

Serves: 10
Time: 1 Hour 15 Minutes

Calories: 90
Protein: 3 Grams
Fat: 25 Grams
Carbs: 13 Grams

INGREDIENTS:

- 2 Tablespoons Olive Oil
- 2 Eggplants, Peeled & Cubed
- 8 Zucchini, Chopped
- 4 Tomatoes, Chopped
- ¼ Cup Basil, Chopped
- 4 Thyme Sprigs
- 2 Yellow Onions, Diced
- 3 Cloves Garlic, Minced
- 3 Bell Peppers, Chopped
- 1 Bay Leaf
- Sea Salt to Taste

DIRECTIONS:

1. Salt your eggplant and leave it in a strainer.

2. Heat a teaspoon of oil in a Dutch oven, cooking your onions for ten minutes. Season with salt.

3. Mix your peppers in, cooking for five more minutes.

4. Place this mixture in a bowl.

5. Heat your oil and sauté zucchini, sprinkling with salt. Cook for five minutes, and place it in the same bowl.

6. Rinse your eggplant, squeezing the water out, and heat another two teaspoons of oil in your Dutch oven. Cook your eggplant for ten minutes, placing it in your vegetable bowl.

7. Heat the remaining oil and cook your garlic. Add in your tomatoes, thyme sprigs and bay leaves to deglaze the bottom.

8. Toss your vegetables back in, and then bring it to a simmer.

9. Simmer for forty-five minutes, and make sure to stir. Discard your thyme and bay leaf. Mix in your basil and serve warm.

Interesting Facts: Eggplant has a variety of vital vitamins and minerals within it's compound. It is high in folic acid, vitamin C, manganese and vitamin K. It aids weight lose and cognitive function. Eggplant is a great meat replacement in a lasagna!

STUFFED BELL PEPPER

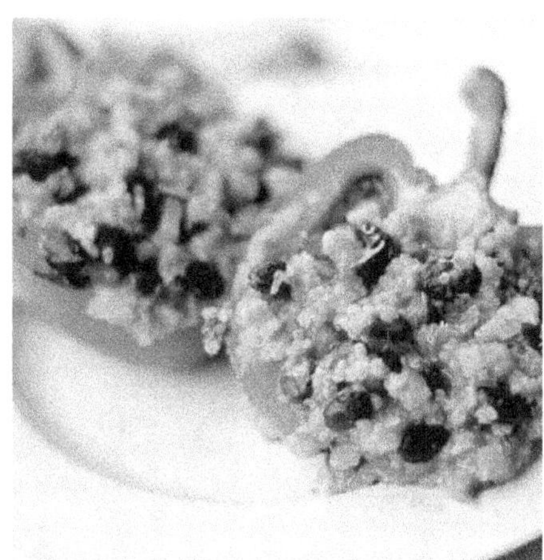

Serves: 4
Time: 25 Minutes

Calories: 126
Protein: 3 Grams
Fat: 5 Grams
Carbs: 19 Grams

INGREDIENTS:

- 4 Bell Peppers, Halved & Hollowed
- ½ Cup Quinoa, Cooked
- 12 Black Olives, Halved
- 1/3 Cup Tomatoes, Sun Dried
- ½ Cup Baby Spinach
- 2 Cloves Garlic, Minced
- Sea Salt & Black Pepper to Taste

DIRECTIONS:

1. Bake your peppers at 400 for ten minutes, and then mix the rest of your ingredients in a bowl.

2. Stuff your peppers with the quinoa mixture.

Interesting Facts: Quinoa: Although it is actually a seed, we treat it mainly as a grain in the way in which it is prepared. This South American gem has an incredible amount of protein and therefore can serve as a great substitute for meat products. Quinoa is an important staple for anyone looking to get the most out of a plant-based diet.

BLACK BEAN BURGERS

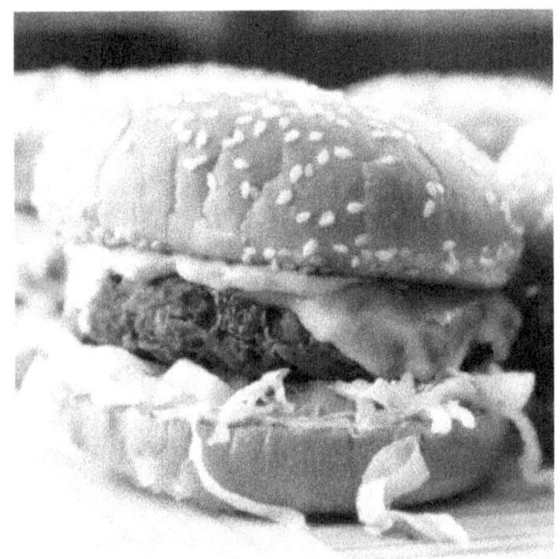

Serves: 6
Time: 25 Minutes

Calories: 173
Protein: 7.3 Grams
Fat: 3.2 Grams
Carbs: 29.7 Grams

INGREDIENTS:

- 1 Onion, Diced
- ½ Cup Corn Nibs
- 2 Cloves Garlic, Minced
- ½ Teaspoon Oregano, Dried
- ½ Cup Flour
- 1 Jalapeno Pepper, Small
- 2 Cups Black Beans, Mashed & Canned
- ¼ Cup Breadcrumbs (Vegan)
- 2 Teaspoons Parsley, Minced
- ¼ Teaspoon Cumin
- 1 Tablespoon Olive Oil
- 2 Teaspoons Chili Powder
- ½ Red Pepper, Diced
- Sea Salt to Taste

DIRECTIONS:

1. Set your flour on a plate, and then get out your garlic, onion, peppers and oregano, throwing it in a pan. Cook over medium-high heat, and then cook until the onions are translucent. Place the peppers in, and sauté until tender.

2. Cook for two minutes, and then set it to the side.

3. Use a potato masher to mash your black beans, and then stir in the vegetables, cumin, breadcrumbs, parsley, salt and chili powder, and then divide it into six patties.

4. Coat each side, and then cook until it's fried on each side.

Interesting Facts: Potatoes are a great starchy source of potassium and protein. They are pretty inexpensive if you are one that is watching their budget. Bonus: Very heart healthy!

FRIED PINEAPPLE RICE

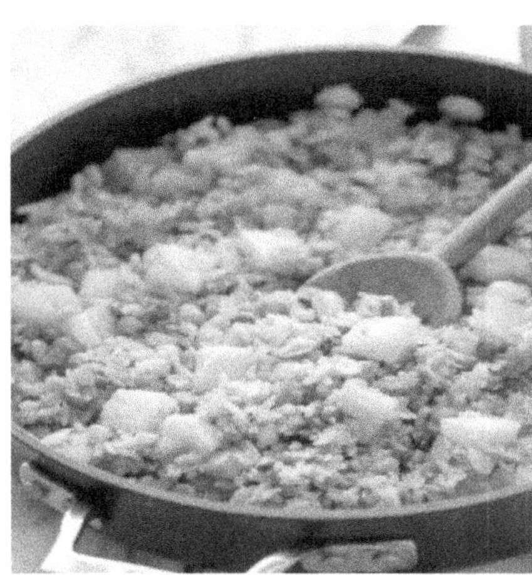

Serves:	6
Time:	30 Minutes
Calories:	179
Protein:	3 Grams
Fat:	4.4 Grams
Carbs:	32.6 Grams

INGREDIENTS:

- 2-3 Cups Brown Rice, Cooked & Cooled
- 1 Tablespoon Sesame Oil
- 2 Tablespoons Raisins (Optional)
- 1 Onion, Small & Chopped
- ½ -3/4 Cup Pineapple, Chopped
- 1 Tablespoon Soy Sauce (Or Braggs Liquid Amino)
- ½ Teaspoon Turmeric
- 1 Tomato, Chopped
- 1 Teaspoon Curry Powder
- 2 Tablespoons Cilantro, Fresh & Chopped
- Sea Salt & Black Pepper to Taste

DIRECTIONS:

1. Start by getting out a sauce pan, and then add your sesame oil to the pan. Sauté your onions until they turn translucent.

2. Add in your cooked rice, soy sauce, pineapple, curry powder and turmeric.

3. Mix well and cook for eight to ten minutes.

4. Serve with cilantro, and season with salt and pepper.

Interesting Facts: _Pineapple:_ This juicy and delicious fruit can be devoured in an array of ways, which means it is a good item to incorporate into meals. Bonus: Since pineapples are full of anti-inflammatory nutrients, they aid in reducing stroke and heart attacks. Double Bonus: Pineapples have also been known to increase fertility!

TOFU POKE

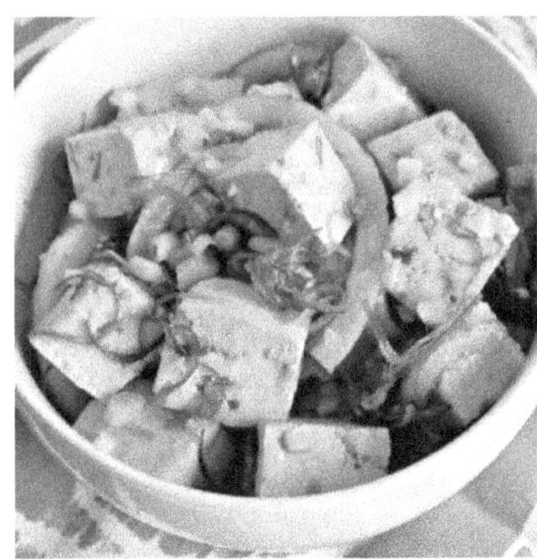

Serves: 4
Time: 30 Minutes

Calories: 262
Protein: 16 Grams
Fat: 15 Grams
Carbs: 19 Grams

INGREDIENTS:

- ¾ Cup Scallions, Sliced Thin
- 1 ½ Tablespoons Mirin
- ¼ Cup Tamari
- 1 ½ Tablespoon Dark Sesame Oil, Toasted
- 1 Tablespoon Sesame Seeds, Toasted (Optional)
- 2 Teaspoons Ginger, fresh & Grated
- ½ Teaspoon Red Pepper, crushed

- 12 Ounces Extra Firm Tofu, Drained & Cut into ½ Inch Pieces
- 4 Cups Zucchini Noodles
- 2 Tablespoons Rice Vinegar
- 2 Cups Carrots, Shredded
- 2 Cups Pea Shoots
- ¼ Cup Basil, Fresh & Chopped
- ¼ Cup Peanuts, Toasted & Chopped (Optional)

DIRECTIONS:

1. Wisk your tamari, mirin, sesame seeds, oil, ginger, red pepper, and scallion greens in a bowl, Set two tablespoons of this sauce aside, and add the tofu to the remaining sauce, Toss to coat,

2. Combine your vinegar and zucchini noodles in a bowl,

3. Divide it between four bowls, topping with tofu, carrots, and a tablespoon of basil and peanuts,

4. Drizzle with sauce before serving,

Interesting Facts: Sesame seeds can be easily added to crackers, bread, salads, and stir-fry meals, Bonus: Help in lowering cholesterol and high blood pressure, Double bonus: Help with asthma, arthritis, and migraines!

Conclusion

There are so many diets in today's society that can be beneficial to our minds, bodies, and health. One of the most popular diets that people transition to is being a vegan. As with any diet you choose, you should consult your doctor and find out if it is safe for you. In this book, we're going to give you vital information about this diet to help give you more information as well. It may be for animal rights, the planet, or maybe they just want to get healthier. Some also have religious, moral, or ethical reasoning behind their decision to be vegan. There are many benefits to adopting this lifestyle but the first thing we need to understand is what is a vegan? A vegan is someone who does not eat or use animal products. This means you need to cut out a lot of things you take for granted such as milk, eggs, cheese, honey, butter and more. Of course, one of the obvious things about a vegan diet is no meat of any kind. You'll have to rethink your dairy, meal plans, even the makeup and clothes you wear or the shampoo you use for your hair. This means you will have to either keep them out altogether from your life or replace them with vegan-friendly options. With so many people turning toward veganism, it's been said that it's turned into a movement by many articles and even some news stations, companies are listening and making amazing new products that are vegan-friendly thereby making it easier than ever to adopt this lifestyle and reap the benefits.

There is really only one way to be a vegan as opposed to other diets where they have subsections and other variations. However, while the definition of being a vegan is solid, there are many different ways to exact a vegan diet. Many have pros and cons and it's up to you to determine which one is the best for your issues and health. It's also important to do your research because some of the diets that claim to be vegan are not because they add meat and dairy into the diet later on after the first few weeks. This is obviously not a vegan diet and therefore not recommended for the changes you're trying to make in your lifestyle.

Some of the most popular vegan diets that people have either been wanting to try or have been curious about are the 'raw till four diet' which has been made amazingly popular due to a vegan on a viral video site. As of now, I believe there is a following of about eight thousand or more, plant-based vegan. Most of the people that use this diet have said that they've tried others, and this was the best for them; low carb vegan such as keto or paleo; and the engine two diets on the opposite side of keto. Some prefer high carb low-fat diets, the detox vegan diet, or even the junk food vegan diet which they love because it proves that being a vegan doesn't have to just stick to healthy 'boring' food but instead can eat amazingly tasty food as well.

One of the most obvious benefits of veganism is that they tend to be skinnier and able to better maintain a healthier weight than most meat eaters. As with any diet, this depends on what you eat. There are many meat and cheese substitutes that are vegan, but some can be high in calories and other things that can make you gain weight if that's all you're eating or junk food related items. Many companies are understanding that more people are becoming vegan and therefore want to put out substitutes and many people fill up on these because they don't do the proper research as to how they should be eating. This causes weight gain. Another problem for new vegans is they listen to fad diet people. An example of this is viral video sites. A lot of the information from these videos is solid and well informed; others, not so much.

There have been people on these channels telling people to eat over five thousand calories a day in fruit and only to exercise an hour. Obviously, this may not be the best advice because that's far too much sugar and calories with only one hour of exercise. You wouldn't be able to burn off that many calories with so little work out time. This could make you balloon up and have a host of health issues. Another fad diet that has come under scrutiny is the 'raw till four' simply because nutritionists have said it's dangerous especially if you're following some of the people on these viral video sites especially when they take it to some of the far extremes. So it's important to know what it is you're doing with your diet. Eating properly can make a vegan skinnier; eating improperly will not.

Since you will no longer be eating meat or dairy, you are likely to be eating foods with a lot less saturated fat. Saturated fat is linked to high cholesterol and increased risk of heart disease. Lower blood pressure is another great benefit of cutting animal products out of your life.

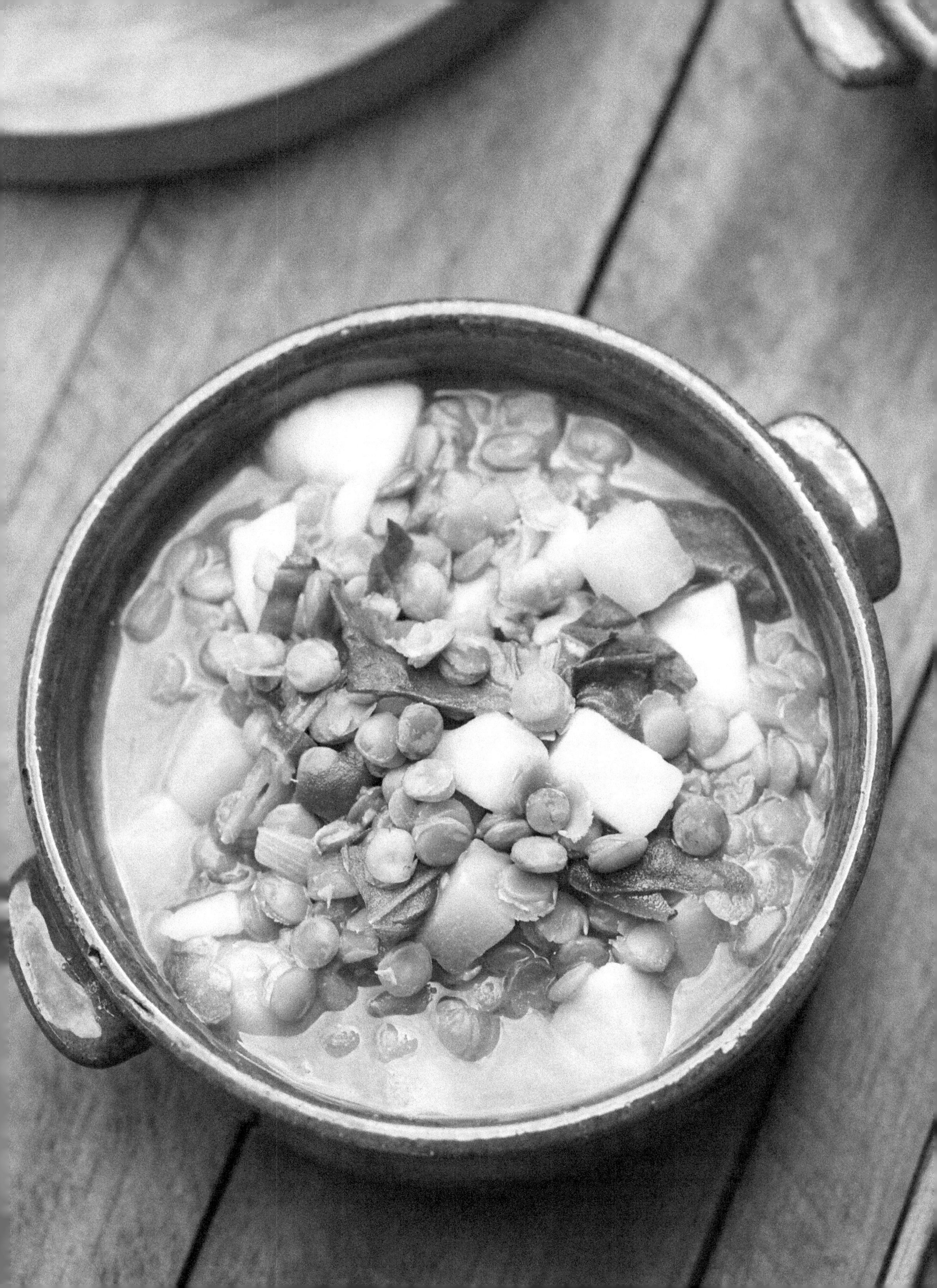

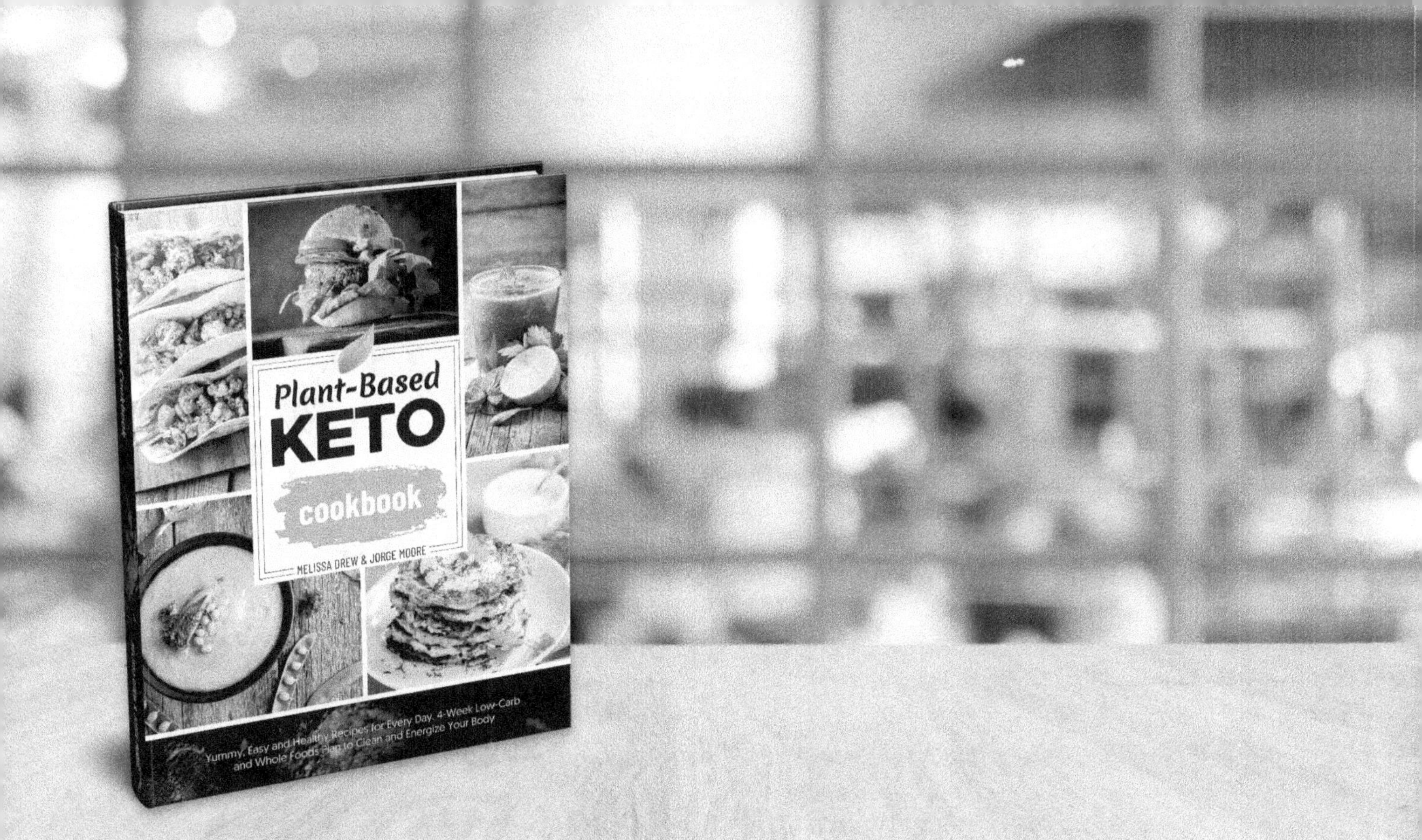

Plant-Based Keto Cookbook

Yummy, Easy and Healthy Recipes for Every Day.
4-Week Low-Carb and Whole Foods Plan
to Clean and Energize Your Body

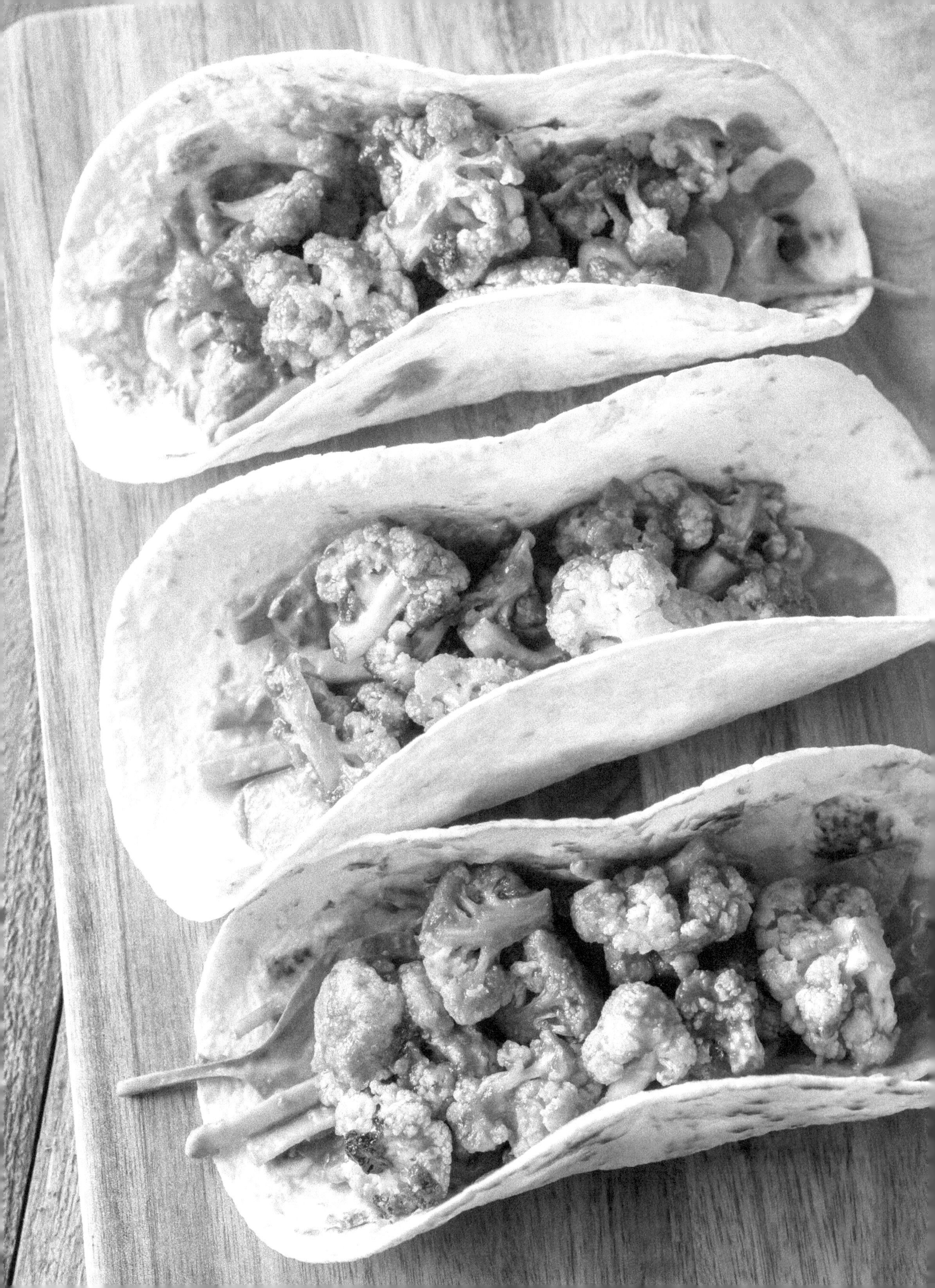

TABLE OF CONTENTS

Book Description **127**

Introduction **129**

Chapter 1: Ketosis, Intermittent Fasting, Macros, and its Benefits **131**

Starting A Ketogenic Diet.. 133
How Weight Loss Is Achieved in General?.. 135
Intermittent Fasting and Weight Loss Through a Caloric Deficit 136

Chapter 2: Foods to Avoid During Plant-Based Diet **139**

Foods to Limit 139
Foods to Avoid 141

Chapter 3: Dealing with Cravings (What to Do When We Feel Cravings) **145**

Tips And Tricks For Handling Carb Cravings... 147
Food to avoid during sugar detox period 150

Chapter 4: Foods to Eat During a Plant-Based Keto Diet **151**

Fruits.. 151
Vegetables 153
Legumes 154
Whole Grains 155

Chapter 5: 30-day Meal Plan **157**

Day 1.. 159
Day 2.. 163
Day 3.. 167
Day 4.. 171
Day 5.. 175
Day 6.. 179
Day 7.. 183
Day 8.. 187

Day 9 191

Day 10 195

Day 11 199

Day 12 203

Day 13 207

Day 14 211

Day 15 215

Day 16 219

Day 17 223

Day 18 227

Day 19 231

Day 20 235

Day 21 239

Day 22 243

Day 23 247

Day 24 251

Day 25 255

Day 26 259

Day 27 263

Day 28 267

Day 29 271

Day 30 275

Chapter 6: Maintaining a progress journal **279**

Conclusion **283**

Book Description

The book is conceptualized with the idea of offering you a comprehensive view of a plant-based diet and how it can benefit the body. You may find the shift sudden, especially if you are a die-hard fan of non-vegetarian items. But, you need not give up anything that you love. Eat everything in moderation.

As you start making the transition to a plant-based diet, you will find some remarkable changes within your body. You will have a better digestive system, and you can control chronic problems. All of these changes will make you happy in the long run. A plant-based diet alone can do wonders, but don't forget to exercise along with this diet to get the best results.

From the recipes and facts that are provided with them, it is proven that plant-based diet mainly consists of ingredients which are generally good for the health. Moreover, most of the nutritional benefits of the ingredients used in the recipes provide similar functionalities and benefits to our health. The most common and repeated benefits are lowering the risk of cancers and provide antioxidants to the body. This would further approve the fact that plant-based diet is an ideal diet for people who would like to transition from regular diet to plant-based as it contains almost similar nutrition with the regular diet plan.

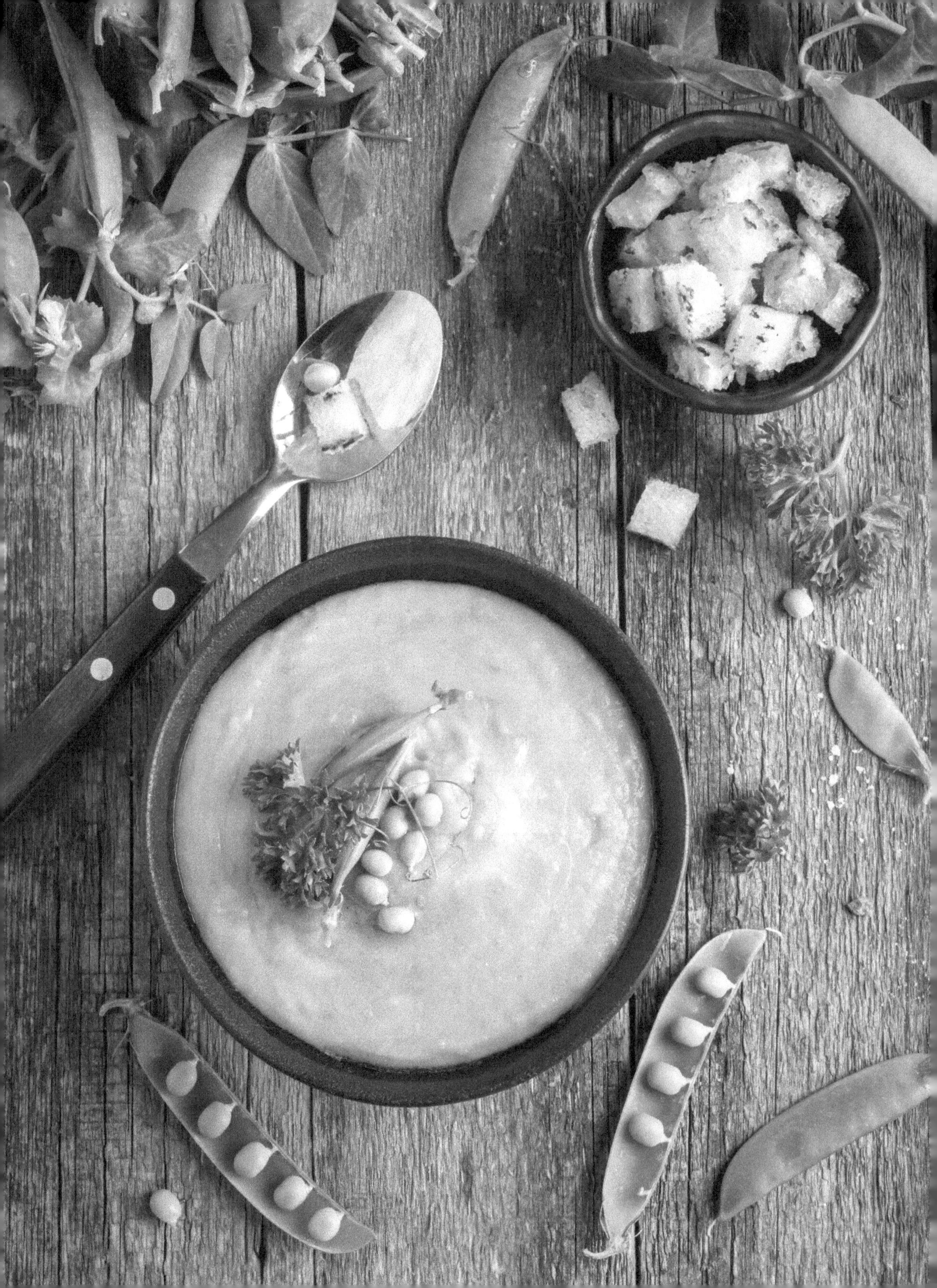

Introduction

A fun way to get yourself used to this new lifestyle is to experiment with different recipes that sound good to you. You'll either realize that you like it and want to eat it again or maybe share it with the people around you if you live with others. Or maybe, instead, you'll be able to tell that it's something you don't like and wouldn't want to try again. Or maybe, it's just something you didn't like cooking. In that case, if you liked the dish but didn't like the work it took to prepare it, which happens to many people, that might lead you to a new restaurant that has the foods you can eat, and you might like how they prepare it. Once you begin experimenting and getting comfortable making the meals, it will become easier to adopt a new diet and find new foods that you like.

You can alter the recipes you already have and use on a daily basis too. If you eat meals with meat, make them vegetarian and then make them vegan before final making them ketogenic or Keto for short. You're still eating a meal that you already enjoy, it is just a different version of it. This can help you with your transition because it's just adapting things you're already used to. An example would be chili. Chili doesn't have to include meat at all, but if you really want it, try a meat substitute. Since beans aren't good for ketogenic because most of them are high in carbs, be sure to go through those carefully looking into the carb content and find a better option for that part of the diet as well. You could come up with an amazing recipe no one ever thought of before or you might be willing to try recipes that you wouldn't before this.

As you adapt to this lifestyle more and more, you should be able to stay on it much easier. Some good tips for maintaining your vegan lifestyle is if you like to eat out, it's like we said it can be difficult with your eating needs. So find out in advance where you can and can't go.

Have special food you can take with you when you leave your house. More and more places are trying to accommodate people's needs but some just don't have everything that you are able to eat because your diet can be a little bit restrictive. This is really going to help you keep yourself from being tempted by other's influence or choices or if a place you're at can't meet the needs of your diet. When you're out at social situations, it can be tempting to get out of your diet or eat foods you know you shouldn't. We have all been there. You can be at a dinner with a few friends and they want to share an appetizer and you think one won't hurt, or they want to drink so you figure one drink won't have too many carbs or something along those lines. A quick tip though; a lot of drinks do have carbs and on a ketogenic diet, it is really not recommended because you'll bust straight through your numbers. Some people even give in to the peer pressure because their friends get upset that someone is not eating like the rest of them. Ignore the peer pressure and do what you want to do. You don't have to answer to anyone but yourself.

Getting support will help you be able to stick to your diet as well. Having people around that love you and support you can be a very big help during this transition. Family can be a big help when you're making such a drastic change. If you are not able to be around encouraging people, then be sure to find motivation and encourage yourself. Too many diets come with negativity and people making fun of others for trying something different. If this is what happens to you, I am sorry because no one deserves that at all and it can be very painful for someone to have to go through. The best thing you can do is ignore the hate and keep a positive attitude and remember what you're doing this for. You're doing this for you, not them, and you don't need their negativity. Ignore it and brush it off and stick to what you really want. I know it can be difficult but just remember you don't need to keep that negativity around you and you are stronger than they are. You are the one that lives your life and you should be happy. Remember this and just keep pushing through. I recommend a reward for you as well. For instance, if you managed to stay a vegan ketogenic for a month, reward yourself with something you've been wanting, like a new pair of shoes or a movie that you've wanted to see. The act of giving yourself a reward will send a positive vibe to your brain that will reinforce your healthy habits and help you to want to keep going on your journey.

Chapter 1:

Ketosis, Intermittent Fasting, Macros, and its Benefits

The benefit of Ketogenic diet is that, it targets fat deposit in the most difficult parts of the body, most especially the abdominal region, thighs and the upper chest areas. Starving yourself may not help cut fat in the most difficult regions, even when you lose fat in such areas, they may return quickly, but this is not the case with Ketogenic diets. Losing weight around your mid-section and around vital organs is necessary in order to avoid serious fat-related diseases.

Ketogenic diets increase the amount of HDL cholesterols while reducing LDL cholesterol levels. Choosing the right type of unsaturated fats in your Ketogenic diet will help increase good cholesterols (HDL cholesterols), and these are healthy for the heart and general wellbeing. Ketogenic diets also help regulate blood sugar levels while reducing the risks of insulin intolerance. When carbs are broken down, they release sugar into the blood quickly and this increases blood sugar rapidly, a condition that triggers more supply of Insulin hormones, but when Ketogenic diets replace high carb diets, less sugar are released slowly into the body, a situation that can stabilize the secretion of Insulin hormones.

Ketogenic diet was coined out of the word "Ketosis", a process whereby the body breaks down more fat into fatty acids and ketones. The breakdown of more fats and ketones will provide sufficient energy sources for the body. Free fatty acids and ketones are simultaneously released in into the body during ketogenic breakdown, these are then made available for the body to burn as fuel.

Normally, the body relies on Glucose as the main source of energy, however, glucose is released when the body breaks down carbs, but the bad side of relying on glucose for energy is that, it can be readily stored as fat in fat cells, organs and tissues, when the energy is not used up. On the other hand, starving the body of glucose will force it to use stored fat in your organs as a source of fuel, even before they are stored for too long inside the body. With the burning of more ketones and fatty acids, there will be less glucose in the body to burn and the body will rapidly adjust to ketogenic phase of deriving energy.

You need to have it in mind that the body can only burn the source of energy present, therefore, constantly consuming ketogenic diet will make fats and proteins readily available as source of energy, as opposed to carbs. Ketogenic diets are effective in two ways, first, they create a net balance of energy in the body, and secondly, they rapidly fill you up (increase satiety), thus, you consume much less than necessary.

With Ketogenic diet, you have to avoid or limit your consumption of carbs to less than 5% of your daily dietary intake. Secondly, you need to avoid unhealthy carbs such as tubers, starches, sugar and other processes foods.

How does Ketogenic diet help you lose weight?

What your body is designed to eat will definitely affect whether you lose weight or not. The earliest humans often rely on what they get during hunting to survive, these include; edible foods, fish and meat, with little or no starch or carb, and that is one of the reasons why they stay slimmer and healthier. With the discovery of processed foods in the modern world (including pasta, white bread and sugary drinks), our bodies have been re-constructed to adjust to such unhealthy lifestyles.

One problem with most starch and sugar is that they can be converted into simple sugars that can be absorbed readily in the blood stream, and the effect of this is that there is a rapid increase in blood sugar level, a condition that triggers a sharp increase in the secretion of Insulin hormones, and this increases the risk of developing diseases such as diabetes type II through rapid weight gain and obesity.

One problem with carbs and sugars is that they increase your cravings, while Ketogenic diet helps you feel fuller quickly and reduce them. You can be at a dinner with a few friends and they want to share an appetizer and you think one won't hurt, or they want to drink so you figure one drink won't have too many carbs or something along those lines. A quick tip though; a lot of drinks do have carbs and on a ketogenic diet, it is really not recommended because you'll bust straight through your numbers. Some people even give in to the peer pressure because their friends get upset that someone is not eating like the rest of them. The early men consume more of ketogenic diets, and that is why they consume much less but get more energy for hunting expenditures. Ketogenic diets help lower your body's reliance on insulin hormones, and then makes it easier for the body to use up its fat reservoir as a source of energy.

You don't have to starve yourself to enjoy the benefits of Ketogenic diet, likewise, there is no need to start counting those calories.

Starting A Ketogenic Diet

Starting out on any new diet can be hard, but a ketogenic diet can be one of the hardest to start. This is because it is a sudden change to a completely different way of eating. Carbs are everywhere and we are programmed to eat as many as we can, so most of us have not had a carb-free day in our entire lives. For this reason, regardless of whether we are starting by reducing our carbs, or going cold turkey, the first few days need to be as easy as possible.

Make sure that you have got rid of all your high carb foods. Some people may do this by eating them all over a week leading up to the first day. Others may throw or give the food away to remove temptation. Either way, you need it gone before you start your diet, to remove all the foods that are likely to make you give up. For this reason, ask other people to keep their carby foods away as well, to prepare your own meals, and to refuse invitations to eat out for a while.

Make sure you have all the foods you will want to eat at home. Check out our recipes nearer the end of the book for an idea of what you will want to have. But the priority is a lot of leafy greens, low carb root vegetables, healthy fats, and lean proteins. If you can, try making meals in advance and freezing them in individual tuppers. And make sure to get some low carb, high fat, high protein snacks, like peanut butter, beef jerky, or boiled eggs. That way you can always have something quick to eat when you need it.

When starting out on a ketogenic diet, you will want to begin with foods you already like. Liver, kale, and almond butter are wonderful additions to a ketogenic diet, but eating things you don't like is not the best way to start a long-term diet. Instead, look through the recipe lists for recipes with foods you love, so that you can truly enjoy your diet.

Next, you will want to start on a morning, when you are not going to work. Stress makes us crave carbs more, and eating carbs is what starts the hunger cycle in the first place. You can be at a dinner with a few friends and they want to share an appetizer and you think one won't hurt, or they want to drink so you figure one drink won't have too many carbs or something along those lines. A quick tip though; a lot of drinks do have carbs and on a ketogenic diet, it is really not recommended because you'll bust straight through your numbers. Some people even give in to the peer pressure because their friends get upset that someone is not eating like the rest of them. So if we start with an empty stomach, running on ketones from the previous night, and we are going to have a relaxed day or two, we will be able to stick it out through the first few days. This massively improves our chances of success, as the first days are the hardest.

When you start a ketogenic diet, you will find many side effects. Most of them are harmless and just part of your body recovering from a lifetime on a high carb diet. Carb cravings are the most common symptom. We have already discussed why these happen, so it is important to remain calm and try and push through. In the next chapter we will offer some solutions for these hunger pangs, but remember that they are at their worst for only a few days, and after that they will be gone.

Indigestion can occur when you first start a ketogenic diet. This is due to a common mistake people make, assuming that this diet is low in all plants. That is not true. On this diet you will eat large amounts of high fibre, low carb plant foods, fatty fruits like avocado, and nuts and seeds. If you do not eat enough fibre you will find that your meals cause reflux, indigestion, and gut cramping. If you are eating plenty of plants but still suffering reflux, indigestion, and gut cramping, consider eliminating dairy from your diet. Sometimes following a ketogenic diet can make an underlying cow milk protein allergy come to the surface. You always would have had this allergy, but it would have been masked by other aspects of your diet.

Finally, if you suffer stomach cramps, diarrhoea, or oily, black stools, then you are eating too much fat. How is it possible to eat too much fat on a low carb, high fat diet? The same way it is possible to pour too much water into a glass. When we are following a ketogenic diet we are using fat as fuel. But we can only absorb so much fat in one go, and burn so much fat. You can be at a dinner with a few friends and they want to share an appetizer and you think one won't hurt, or they want to drink so you figure one drink won't have too many carbs or something along those lines. A quick tip though; a lot of drinks do have carbs and on a ketogenic diet, it is really not recommended because you'll bust straight through your numbers. Some people even give in to the peer pressure because their friends get upset that someone is not eating like the rest of them. When we eat more fat than we can absorb, our bodies just let it pass through us. This is largely harmless, but has the side effect of damaging our gut bacteria, one of the exact things we are trying to fix without diet. So if you notice these side effects, start reducing your fat intake until your stools return to normal.

Besides these symptoms, you should also experience a whole host of beneficial symptoms. Some of the most beneficial symptoms, like an improvement in metabolism, and weight loss, will take longer to happen. But others happen within days. You will find your appetite begins to come under your control. As your insulin spikes and crashes disappear, your body gets used to having a steady supply of energy. This means that rather than feeling hungry every single time your blood sugar drops, and snacking between meals, you are eating a healthy meal and going straight through to the next one without feeling hungry.

You will find that yeast infections and skin conditions improve, or even disappear entirely. This is because your candida is not being fed, so it has nothing to grow from. You can be at a dinner with a few friends and they want to share an appetizer and you think one won't hurt, or they want to drink so you figure one drink won't have too many carbs or something along those lines. A quick tip though; a lot of drinks do have carbs and on a ketogenic diet, it is really not recommended because you'll bust straight through your numbers. Some people even give in to the peer pressure because their friends get upset that someone is not eating like the rest of them. Candida causes many types of yeast infection, and several types of skin problem, being the root cause of most cases of dandruff, for starters. It also makes other conditions, like eczema, worse, by irritating the skin and growing under and around dead skin cells.

You will find your moods are more even. That "hangry" feeling you get when your blood sugar drops are not normal. It is your body responding to a lack of glucose, trying to get you to eat carbs. At first you may feel the carb-hungry anger more intensely than usual, but after a couple of days your body gets used to not having those constant spikes and crashes in blood sugar. No energy crashes mean no cravings, means no eating carbs, means no spikes, means no more crashes. It is vitally important to fight this cycle and restore order, even if you have no intention of following a ketogenic diet for life.

How Weight Loss Is Achieved in General?

Before we look at the best way that you can use intermittent fasting to help you reduce your body fat percentage, let's first quickly consider how weight loss generally works – think of this as the science behind effective and guaranteed weight loss.

When you eat something – regardless of what it is – it means you are putting calories into your body. Nutrients are broken down and absorbed by your body, while carbohydrates are broken down and then processed into glucose, which is then distributed through your body to provide cells with energy.

When excess glucose is present in your body, it will usually be stored as fat cells through a rather complicated process that we are not going to be discussing in detail here. As fat cells increase, you gain weight – ultimately leading to you becoming overweight and then slowly obese.

Now, on the other hand, when you are physically active – whether you are walking, dancing, or going hard on the treadmill at the gym – you are burning calories. Your body uses more glucose for energy, and when the reserves run out, the body starts looking toward stored fat cells in order to generate more energy. This energy then allows you to continue running on that treadmill or allows you to pick up the set of weights a few more times.

So, to sum this up – you eat, you gain calories; you exercise, you lose calories.

When the number of calories you eat surpasses the number of calories you lose, then you gain weight. Think of this within a 24-hour cycle. If you eat 2,000 calories, but only burn 1,000, then you gain weight to the value of those extra 1,000 calories that are left behind at the end of the day.

When you eat more calories than you burn, it means there is a caloric surplus. You are gaining weight and cannot lose weight with this strategy.

To lose weight, this entire equation needs to be in an opposite manner. You need to lose more calories than you burn. If you eat food that calculates to around 2,000 calories each day, you need to burn more than the 2,000 calories if you wish ever to see your fat go away and the number of the scale go down.

When your daily calorie intake is less than the number of calories you lose, then it means you have a caloric deficit – this is the ideal goal that you are striving toward when you are aiming to reduce your body weight.

Intermittent Fasting and Weight Loss Through a Caloric Deficit

With intermittent fasting, you still need to create a caloric deficit. I've seen some people think that simply because they are fasting, they will lose weight, regardless of the other factors in their life. This is not true.

No matter how beneficial fasting might be and a program that utilizes intermittent fasting, you will still need to take the science behind weight loss into account. If your caloric intake is more than how many calories you lose in a day, then you set the way for weight gain and not weight loss.

Intermittent fasting can make things a little easier, however. It has been found that people who follow an intermittent fasting program eventually experience improvements in their level of satiety. Their appetite is reduced, in other words. Since weight gain often lies within the fact that a person is unable to control their urges to eat inappropriate times, the reduced appetite will certainly be beneficial.

Additionally, because all meals of the day need to be squeezed into an eight-hour window with the particular intermittent fasting method that I am focusing on in this guide, it usually means that you will still feel somewhat full with your second meal after you had your first. When the time comes to have your third meal, the second meal will still be satisfying your appetite a little. You'll end up not wanting to overload your plate every chance you get – this means it becomes much, much easier than before to be in control of how many calories you will be consuming on a day-to-day basis.

Now, combine this with exercise. You won't even have to hit the gym too hard and may even be able to burn an adequate number of calories exercising at home if you are able to reduce the number of calories you consume by simply feeling full from the last meal when the time for the next meal comes.

Chapter 2:

Foods to Avoid During Plant-Based Diet

Now, we get to the fun part! If you still believe that a plant-based diet is going to be restrictive, be prepared to have your mind changed forever. The truth is, the plant-based diet includes a wide variety of foods that you get to enjoy. I know so many people who enjoy this diet and the benefits that go along with it; isn't it about time you join them?

To start off, we'll go over all of the incredible foods that you'll be enjoying. After that, we'll go in depth on the foods you should avoid on the plant-based diet. As mentioned earlier, there's a misconception that plant-based means no meat. That's wrong. You can still have the meat. However, after reading about the troubles it can cause to your health and our dear planet, you might want to limit it or even give it a miss. Once you have everything you need to know, be sure to read the next chapter where I've created an expandable grocery list for you, some delicious recipes and even a simple meal plan to help you get started. I want to give you as much help as possible so success is closer than you think in your plant-based journey.

Foods to Limit

In this next section, I will list off the foods you should still eat, but in sparing amounts. This means that even though they're allowed and do provide great health benefits, it doesn't mean you should eat them every day. That's because they also add a high amount of fat into your diet. This is especially crucial if you're looking to lose weight.

- Avocado

I said the same thing you're probably saying to yourself right now: Avocado is a fruit? Indeed, it is, but they are very different from your typical fruit. While most fruits are high in carbohydrate, avocado is low in carbs and acts more as an excellent source of healthy fats. The nutrients found in avocado include monounsaturated fat and oleic acid, both of which research has shown to be associated with better heart health and reduced inflammation.

- Nuts & Nut Butters

They are also commonly used as a healthy snack option. However, they do contain a relatively high fat content. The fat found in nuts include monounsaturated fat, omega-6, and omega-3 polyunsaturated fat. It should be noted that these fats are considered healthy, but you'll still want to consume them in moderation.

Examples: Peanut Butter, Tahini. Cashew Butter, Almond Butter, Walnuts, Pistachios, Pecans, Peanuts, Coconut, Cashews, Almonds.

- Seeds & Seed Butters

Just like nuts; seeds are a great snacking alternative. Seeds are extremely nutritious and are an excellent source of fiber. They could potentially help to lower your blood pressure, cholesterol levels, and blood sugar. However, it's true that there can be too much of a good thing. So, although seeds contain polyunsaturated fats and healthy monounsaturated fats, which are essentially good fats, they should still be limited. Examples: Sunflower Seeds, Sesame Seeds, Flaxseeds, Chia Seeds.

- Beverages

It should be noted that water is going to be the best beverage for you, but it is completely understandable if you don't want to just drink water for the rest of your life. This is why the following beverages are allowed, but should be limited to only a few times per week.

- Fruit Juices

- Unsweetened Plant Milk, eg. Soy Milk or Almond Milk

- Processed Smoothies

- Soy Yogurt

- Dried Fruits

Dried fruits are more processed compared to their whole or raw versions. If you do include dried fruits in your diet, you'll want to make sure that they are unsulfured. Some examples of dried fruits you could try include: Raisins, Medjool Dates, Currants, Cherries, Blueberries, Apricots, or Apples.

- Sweeteners

Adding a little sweetener is the secret ingredient to making yummy desserts or to satisfy your sweet tooth. However, you'll want to choose those that are minimally processed. I suggest looking for maple sugar, date sugar, or even cane sugar. On top of these options, you can always choose pure maple syrup. The goal is to make sure that you're getting real maple syrup and not something that is maple-flavored. These are very important differences you'll want to be conscious of when you start a plant-based diet.

- Condiments

When it comes to condiments, you'll need to be selective as well. While there are plenty of options on the market, you'll still want to select condiments that are going to be compliant with your new diet. Some of my favorites include Hot Sauce, Wasabi Paste, Vegan Worcestershire Sauce, Apple Cider Vinegar and Tomato Sauce. In the next chapter, you'll be gifted with a thorough grocery list to help you get started on your new diet!

Foods to Avoid

Here is where it might get tough for some of you. It is important to remember this phrase: "do not let the food control you." You are in control. You are the only person who can decide what goes into your body. The question is this, "do you want to fuel your body with nutrients or clog it up with unhealthy foods?" While it may take some work at first, you'll soon get used to it and naturally avoid these foods!

- Animal-based Foods

This is a given but remember that it isn't absolutely restricted! You SHOULD avoid them, but if you feel you absolutely need an animal protein, it is allowed in small portions. Some of the animal-based proteins you should avoid include fish, shellfish, game meats, chicken, turkey, pork, lamb, and beef. We have already gone over why meat might not be the best for your health, so how much of it you would allow in your diet is a decision you'll have to make for yourself.

- Eggs

This is another food that is tough for some people at the beginning. You'd be surprised to know that eggs are included in so many different types of foods. Whether it's your favorite bread or muffin, you'll want to avoid eggs (egg whites included). While it may be difficult in the beginning, it is absolutely possible to avoid them. So don't give in.

- Dairy

You'll want to avoid dairy while on the plant-based diet. This includes foods such as cream, yogurt, butter, cheese, and milk. You'll also need to be mindful of any food that contains a dairy product, or an ingredient made from a dairy product. As long as it is coming from an animal, like sheep, goats or cows, it should be avoided. Luckily, there're plenty of plant-based alternatives to keep you satisfied. Some examples are soymilk, cashew cheese, tofu yogurt, coconut whipped cream and frozen banana ice cream!

- Artificial & Refined Foods

Remember that this diet is all about consuming foods that are plant-based. From this point on, you will want to avoid foods that contain chemical additives such as preservatives, flavorings, or colorings. You'll also want to avoid any foods that have refined sugars or bleached flour. In the tips and tricks chapter, you'll be learning everything you need to know about reading a food label to help you avoid these ingredients. It can be tricky at first, but with some effort, you can say goodbye to artificial foods forever.

- Oils

If you are looking to lose weight, this is going to be a big factor for you! When you follow a plant-based diet, you'll be saying goodbye to any type of extracted oils. This includes fish oil, coconut oil, vegetable oil, and even olive oil! Don't worry, you'll soon find out once you get into the recipes section in the next chapter!

I understand this might be a lot to take in at once right now and I don't blame you if you feel a bit overwhelmed. However, I'm determined to provide you this information so as to give you a head start. By now, you should've understood the gist of it – whole foods are good; artificial foods are bad. The essential nutrients we need are found in both animals and plants, so why not choose the one that comes from plants?

One of the first questions I asked myself when I stumbled upon the plant-based diet was, "how is this diet going to be any different from the rest?" It is an important question as there're so many different diets on the market nowadays. Each diet claims to save your life, get rid of your disease and help you lose weight. At the end of the day, although not every diet is for everyone, you can never go wrong with being more conscious of what you eat.

The plant-based diet puts an emphasis on eating both fresh and whole ingredients. Basically, you are going to want to avoid food that has been highly processed. By eating minimally processed foods and increasing the plants in your diet, it will be effective in helping you to lose weight, improve your health, or both!

While there is no true definition to a plant-based diet, it is so much more than a diet. Most diets set you up for failure. If you're anything like me, you must have tried a handful of them already. Many individuals follow strict rules like cutting sugar, cutting carbs, or completely eliminating food groups that they love. Unfortunately, it's hard to do it this way because it's hard to just drop your bad habits. On the other hand, a plant-based diet doesn't have strict rules like these. Instead, it has basic principles that anyone can follow on their own time and pace. The best part is that it is inclusive, so you can make this lifestyle a family event!

Often times, a plant-based diet is confused with a vegan or vegetarian diet. The plant-based diet is the umbrella term where veganism and vegetarianism falls under. A plant-based diet is extremely versatile to help fit the needs of a variety of people. Yes, there is an emphasis on whole foods that have been minimally processed, but technically, animal products are still allowed on this diet, though they should be limited!

You'll be encouraged to learn how to enjoy new types of food such as nuts, seeds, legumes, whole grains, fruits, and vegetables. Later in the chapters of this book, you'll even be provided with a grocery list, meal plan, and the foods you should avoid and the foods you should enjoy. As I said, I'm setting you up for complete success here! When we do this together, we'll also be able to save our planet one healthy person at a time.

Of course, thinking about moving to this diet is going to be your first step. While it sounds like an excellent idea, often times it is difficult to know where to start.

Chapter 3:

Dealing with Cravings
(What to Do When We Feel Cravings)

Food has strong associations with memories, good times, and even love. There may be certain foods you've adored since childhood that are now out of reach because they are high in refined carbohydrates. These foods, strongly associated with comfort, tradition, and memories, may have an emotional pull that is difficult to resist.

Along with an emotional connection to food, there may be physical reasons for cravings, as well. If you've followed the Standard American Diet (SAD) most of your life, eating macronutrient ratios according to the USDA's food pyramid, then you've probably been eating a lot of refined carbohydrates. Foods high in refined carbohydrates can actually be addicting, according to a 2013 study from Boston Children's Hospital published in **Medscape Medical News**.

With that emotional connection, as well as a potential physical addiction to certain foods, it's understandable that cravings arise—even when you've made the choice to eliminate those foods from your life. The trick, then, becomes finding ways to manage these cravings while maintaining your healthy new lifestyle.

THE LOW-CARB LIFESTYLE

Choosing a low-carb lifestyle isn't a temporary solution to weight or health issues. Instead, it is a lifelong commitment to your health. Long-term success depends upon continued carbohydrate restriction. However, to realistically maintain the diet for a lifetime, you also need some sensible recipes that allow you to eat the foods you crave and still stay on plan.

Most diets provide tips and direction on how to succeed long-term and maintain weight loss and health gains. For example, the Atkins diet offers several phases that gradually ramp up healthy carb intake. By phase three and four, you move into pre-maintenance and maintenance phases, which allow you to make sensible choices for a lifetime of low-carbohydrate eating. Though you'll eat more carbs in these phases, you still won't be going hog-wild. You'll always need to restrict carbs on some level to maintain results.

By now, you probably have a host of recipes and meals that adhere to the plan's requirements. You know which foods fit your lifestyle and which are best avoided. Still, even with this knowledge and experience, cravings may lurk just around the corner.

Fortunately, there's no need to fall off the low-carb wagon to satisfy those cravings. You can give in a little by choosing modified versions of foods that are lower in carbs than their traditional counterparts. Of course, if you do eat these crave busters, the best way to balance this is to adjust carb counts throughout the rest of the day or week so carb levels stay close to those prescribed by your current eating plan and phase.

The recipes in this book remain very close to your low-carb plan allotments. While slightly higher in carbs than the typical low-carb foods you eat—some with as many as 5 grams of net carbs more than other foods—they aren't going to blow your entire carb budget. Instead of giving in to cravings with the "forbidden" versions of these foods, use these lower-carb versions to indulge, and adjust your remaining carb counts accordingly. Think of it as part of a winning strategy to maintain your healthy-living plan for the long term.

Your detox period will not be smooth, especially during the first days. They may even be worse than you'd expected. If this is your first time, you might be swayed to doubt that you're not doing it right. Doubts that maybe you're missing something. Maybe you ate something you shouldn't have eaten in the first place. You may then be tempted to abort the mission. "This looks like a mission impossible." But look, isn't it through the pain that you will gain? And just like any other road to success struggles and setbacks are involved? Same case here. Remember it can only get better. Your health is taking a step back before leaping forward. And you gonna love it and appreciate the sacrifice.

Just so you may be aware of the common side effects to experience during the detox period, here are some:

- Sporadic sleep, constipation and diarrhea, skin rashes/breakouts, cold-like symptoms, mucus drainage, headaches, low energy/exhaustion, bad breath, gas/bloating, and emotions resurfacing

But your reward is waiting for you. You will start experiencing the goodness of the cleansing even during the period and after. Talk about a clearer skin, better sleep, increased energy, increased sense of taste, fat loss, lower cholesterol, less depression, less bloating, regular bowel movements, and less sugar cravings. And there are many more benefits far much outdoing the sugar related problems.

You will crave that sugar. You will miss that food with refined sugar. The suggested foods herein are not as sweet as the sugars. But remember it is only for a short while and you will not to worry anymore when you see that cake. That honey in the kitchen looking at you like 'eat me please' because this craving will reduce and will have no force to make you have the temptation.

A times cooking might seem to be a time-consuming task. "I should probably grab some food from the shop, perhaps they say it's cooked well and has no sugars." That is not always the case. It is not an assurance either. Do you want to enjoy the full benefits out of the period? Then take time to cook for yourself. You might think that you have no time to cook but there's always time. Only if you plan well ahead. This guide has meal plans and recipes designed to accommodate two people. Probably you have a family member or a friend who needs the detox as you do. Or even more, huh. Working as a team is an added advantage. Encourage one another and together you'll reap the benefits of the period.

Even with this guide in place, you still should have a mindset for success. Sometimes due to unavoidable circumstances, you might miss following a part of the plan. What should you do? Set and discipline yourself to complete the detox period. Temptations are there, in plenty. Your friend's wedding is happening this weekend and you'd promised to attend. Obviously, there will be amazing sugary foods and beverages. "A small bite won't make much difference, will it?" Yes, it will. But there's a way around this temptations, besides the personal discipline. Take time and look for a period you will have no such plans to affect your detox. Plan ahead and you will have no problems.

Tips And Tricks For Handling Carb Cravings.

Carb cravings are one of the hardest parts of cutting your carb intake right back. We have already discussed why our bodies resist going low carb so aggressively, but that is of little comfort to someone who is going through the cravings themselves. Instead, here are some helpful ways of coping with the carb cravings until they naturally pass.

1: Sweeteners.

Although artificial sweeteners are hardly a health tonic, they can make for a very useful tool when controlling our carb cravings. Consider natural forms of sweeteners first, but most of them have a small amount of carbs, so if you will be using a lot, choose artificial ones.

Some people advise against using sweeteners, claiming that they will prolong the psychological addiction to carbs. However, although this is slightly true, it isn't the point. The physical addiction to carbs is far more intense than any psychological addiction, and if we go long enough without too many carbs, that addiction will break. After we have defeated the physical aspect of our addiction we can then consider cutting out sweeteners and fighting the psychological aspect. But until then, sweeteners are very useful.

2: Eat more protein.

Sometimes when we crave carbs we are just plain hungry. After so long eating too many carbs, all day every day, with every meal, our stomach rumbles and carbs are the first thing we try to get to eat. This means that we need to retrain our appetite signals to crave different foods, not just sugars and starches. And the first step to that is eating more protein. Eating protein fills our stomachs and triggers the release of hormones that make us feel satisfied. So if we need calories, protein should help.

3: Fill up on greens.

The annoying part of carb cravings, though, is that because they are so misdirected, they could be a craving for any vital nutrient. If eating protein doesn't satisfy you, then it might be that you need vitamins and minerals. A large green salad, or a low carb stir-fry or soup, will fill your stomach with fibre, and add vital nutrients to your diet. This can take longer to have an effect, so be patient. If it works and you feel better, increase your daily greens intake until you no longer feel cravings.

4: Drink some water.

And if protein and greens both fail, you might actually just be thirsty. When you rarely drink clean, simple water, your body doesn't know how to ask for it. Instead, it will fire up your appetite signals as soon as you get dehydrated. Get a glass of water and drink it quickly. Then get a second glass and sip it over half an hour. This rehydration might make your cravings go away.

5: Go for a walk.

Finally, if nothing hits the spot for your cravings, try and distract yourself. Mental activity can be hard in the middle of carb cravings, and idle distractions like watching television don't really take anything away from it. Instead, try and get moving. A walk around the block, or through some fields, can really take your mind away from cravings. And exercise, at least whilst you're doing it, will help you fight hunger. Just make sure to have a healthy meal ready for when you are done exercising.

6: Meditate.

Mindfulness is a great way of fighting cravings. You know, on a conscious level, that your cravings for carbs are not a vital need, that your body is misleading you, and that the cravings will go away. But your body, your primitive self, does not know that. It is thought that meditation is a way of communicating with your body and cooperating with each other. Some Buddhist monks can sit on solid ice blocks bare naked, or even slow their heart rates right down, without suffering harm, just by meditating and focusing on their bodies.

Food to avoid during sugar detox period

Vegetables

Tapioca, parsnips, boiled carrots, sweet potato, potatoes, French fries, pumpkin, corn

Grains and Refined Carbs

White rice, rye, wheat, brown rice, oats, wild rice, corn, sweet corn, long grain rice, barley, bread, cupcakes, couscous, candy, pasta, bagels, crackers, pizza, breadsticks, pita, croissants, brownies, pastries, English muffin, baguette, corn tortilla, doughnut, waffles, angel food cake, popcorn

Drinks

Sports drinks and almost all sodas and fruit juices

Sugar and snacks

Honey, syrup, candy bars, sugary snacks, sucrose, glucose, jelly beans

Fruits

Watermelon, banana, tangerines, dried dates, raisins

Chapter 4:

Foods to Eat During a Plant-Based Keto Diet

One of the major benefits of the plant-based diet is that you can say goodbye to calorie counting! I mentioned earlier that the foods you'll be eating will be much more calorie-dense, meaning that you'll feel fuller more easily and for a longer time! You can say goodbye to counting calories and hello to actually enjoying your food! To begin, we will go over the foods that you can consume freely.

Fruits

While all fruits are allowed, it should be noted that not all fruits are created equal. Each fruit provides its own unique health benefits and coming right up, you will get my compilation of some of the healthiest fruits for your plant-based diet.

- Cranberries

Cranberries are unique fruits that are rich in vitamin K1, vitamin E, manganese, vitamin C, and copper! They also have a significant number of antioxidants that improve health significantly. Cranberries also contain A-type proanthocyanidins, which research has shown, to be a great help in preventing gum inflammation and urinary tract infections.

- Strawberries

Strawberries are among the most recommended fruits. It is also full of potassium, folate, manganese, and vitamin C. When compared to other fruits, strawberries are considered to have a low glycemic index, meaning they won't cause blood sugar spikes. A study published in the Anticancer Research journal has found that strawberries can actually prevent tumor growth.

- Mango

Mango is an excellent fruit to add to your fruit list, especially in the summertime! Mango has soluble fiber and provides vitamin C, which makes it anti-inflammatory. It also has strong antioxidants that lower the risk of diseases. In animal studies, it was found that the compounds in mangos could help protect against diabetes.

- Pomegranate

If you haven't had pomegranates before, you're missing out! Pomegranates are nutrient dense and have an excellent level of antioxidants to keep you healthy. In fact, a study published in the Journal of Agricultural and Food Chemistry has found that pomegranate juice has 3 times higher levels of antioxidants compared to red wine and green tea! On top of this, it's also full of different kinds of polyphenols, which reduces the chance of developing cancer.

- Apples

We have all heard it, an apple a day keeps the doctor away. As it turns out, there seems to be some truth to the saying! Apples are very nutritious and contain high amounts of vitamin K, potassium, vitamin C, and fiber! They also provide B vitamins. Research has shown that antioxidants found in apples can help promote heart health and may reduce the risk of Alzheimer's, cancer, and type 2 diabetes.

- Blueberries

Blueberries are most commonly known for their high levels of antioxidants, but they are also high in manganese, vitamin K, vitamin C and fiber! Jam-packed with all these nutrients, it's no wonder blueberries can help reduce the risk of certain chronic conditions including diabetes and heart disease.

- Pineapple

With just one cup of this delicious fruit, you receive all of the vitamin C you need for the day, plus a hefty amount of manganese too. Pineapple also has bromelain, which helps to digest proteins. In addition, studies have proven that pineapples can help fight and protect against cancer and tumor growth.

- Grapefruit

The list of fruits you can enjoy goes on and on, but I'll end off with grapefruit. Grapefruit is an excellent source of the vitamins and minerals. Research shows that grapefruit is associated with reduced cholesterol levels and may help prevent the forming of kidney stones.

Vegetables

On a plant-based diet, the bulk of what you'll be eating will be vegetables. Obviously, this does not come as a surprise. There are plenty of vegetables for you to enjoy, but the following are the real powerhouses that you'll want to include as often as possible into your diet.

- Brussels Sprouts

The truth is, it is all in the preparation! Brussels sprouts contain an antioxidant known as kaempferol. This specific antioxidant is linked to the prevention of any cell damage that is caused by oxidative stress, and is an important antioxidant to keep chronic diseases at bay. Additionally, brussels sprouts are an excellent source of potassium, manganese, folate, and vitamin C, A and K!

- Garlic

Rejoice all my garlic lovers! Garlic has many roots in our history as a medicinal plant. One of its main active compounds is allicin, and the research has shown that this compound helps to regulate blood sugar and promotes excellent heart health. It was also found in a study published in The American Journal of Clinical Nutrition that garlic is beneficial in lowering total blood cholesterol, LDL cholesterol, and triglycerides, all while increasing healthy HDL cholesterol.

- Broccoli

It also contains an abundant amount of potassium, manganese, and folate, which we need daily. Broccoli also contains sulforaphane, which has been found to have a protective effect against cancer. In one specific study, sulforaphane was successfully able to reduce the number and size of breast cancer cells while simultaneously blocking tumor growth.

- Carrots

In one cup of carrots, you'll receive 428% of your daily recommended vitamin A. Carrots also contain the antioxidant beta-carotene which is associated with cancer prevention. In fact, one study found that by eating one serving of carrots during a week could lower the risk of prostate cancer by 5%.

- Spinach

Of course, spinach is on the list! Spinach tops the charts as being one of the healthiest vegetables, and it isn't hard to understand why! Spinach is rich in iron, vitamin A, vitamin K, and is also packed with antioxidants. It also contains the compound called carotenoid, which the research has shown, can help individuals reduce their risk of cancer.

Legumes

While beans and legumes are more known for their fiber and B vitamins, they're also the main source of protein for your new, plant-based diet. Now, I will list some of the healthier ones you should make into staples, or when you're looking to switch out those animal proteins.

- Black Beans

Black beans might just become one of your new favorite foods. Not only are they packed with fiber and folate, they also offer 15.2 grams of protein in just one cup! These beans are beneficial as they have a lower glycemic index when compared to other foods with higher carbohydrates content. This means they can help control your blood sugar levels while being eaten as a staple. Scientists have even found evidence that black beans can help individuals manage their weight and type 2 diabetes.

- Kidney Beans

These beans are another food that is fairly common on a plant-based diet. Comparable to black beans, a cup of kidney beans contains an impressive 13.4 grams of protein. They are also high in fiber and are known to help slow down the absorption of sugar into the bloodstream. In the same study mentioned earlier, it was found that there is a connection between kidney beans and type 2 diabetes as well. On top of that, the fiber in kidney beans also helped to reduce the spike in blood sugar after finishing a meal.

- Peas

Peas are an excellent source of protein and fiber. They also have the ability to reduce insulin and blood sugar after a meal. What's more, you're not restricted to just plain peas anymore. Now, there is something called pea starch and it's also good for you. In fact, there is a study from the European Journal of Nutrition that discovered that pea starch could help you feel fuller for a longer amount of time.

- Lentils

In one cup of lentils, you'll get a whopping 17.9 grams of protein! The research has shown that eating lentils helps to reduce blood sugar and lower the risk of diabetes. Another study published in The American Journal of Clinical Nutrition has even shown that lentils can improve gut health by increasing your bowel function. When the stomach is emptied at a quicker rate, digestion increases and spikes in blood sugar is prevented.

- Chickpeas

The final source of protein that makes my list is chickpeas. They are often referred to as garbanzo beans and make an excellent source of fiber and protein. In one cup of chickpeas, you'll get 14.5 grams of protein. Specifically, chickpeas are great for reducing blood sugar levels and increasing sensitivity to insulin. It should also be noted that chickpeas can help improve bowel movement, by reducing the level of bad bacteria stuck in your intestines.

Whole Grains

As you switch to a plant-based diet, grains are going to become another staple in your household. Firstly, there are 3 types of whole grains – the bran, the germ, and the endosperm. Each one of these has its own nutrients, which are vital for your health. Whole grains are excellent as they are high in dietary fiber, B vitamins, selenium, phosphorus, manganese, magnesium, and iron!

- Quinoa

In South America, quinoa is a superfood! This is because this grain is packed with fiber, healthy fats, proteins and all the minerals and vitamins you need for a well-rounded diet. A study has shown that quinoa also contains the antioxidant kaempferol, (just like Brussels sprouts) and it helps in the prevention of certain types of cancers, heart disease and chronic inflammation.

- Brown Rice

For a majority of you, up until this point in your life, you've mostly been eating white rice. Yet, brown rice is the healthier alternative. This is because brown rice is a whole grain – it still has the bran and germ intact, which makes it richer in fiber, antioxidants, minerals, and vitamins. Along with these benefits, brown rice also happens to be gluten-free, which makes it an excellent choice if you need to follow a gluten-free diet.

- Whole-grain Bread

On top of switching from white rice to brown rice, you'll also want to consider switching from white bread to whole-grain bread. There's a wide variety including whole-grain tortillas, bagels, rolls, and rye bread. Although it's a simple switch, you're actually adding more whole grains into your diet and this is extremely nutritious.

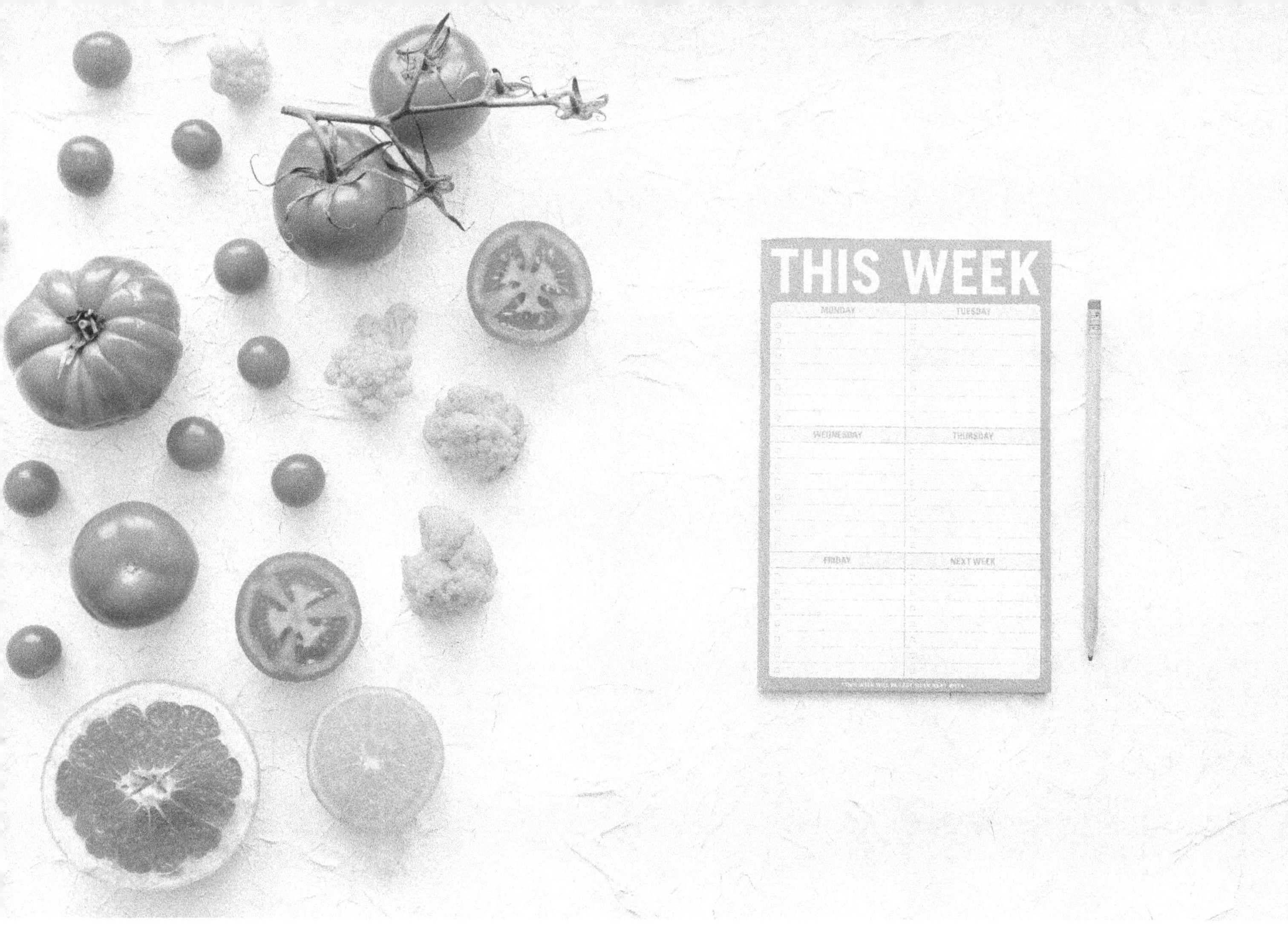

Chapter 5:

30-day Meal Plan

Below you will find 4 weeks' worth of meal plans and a shopping list to accompany it. The list will not have the amounts of the individual food you will need because that will depend on the number of servings. It also doesn't include basic things people normally have in their pantries such as oil, salt, pepper, and ground spices.

To use the meal plan you may use it exactly as is and write out the amount of each item you need or you may switch it up and make your own shopping list.

Day 1

Shopping list

- Chia seeds
- Non-dairy milk
- Natural nut butter of your choice
- Vanilla extract
- Maple syrup
- Tomatoes
- Cucumbers
- Onion
- Parsley
- Salt and pepper
- Virgin olive oil
- Balsamic vinegar
- Brown rice
- Lemon
- Vinegar
- Oregano

BREAKFAST RECIPE

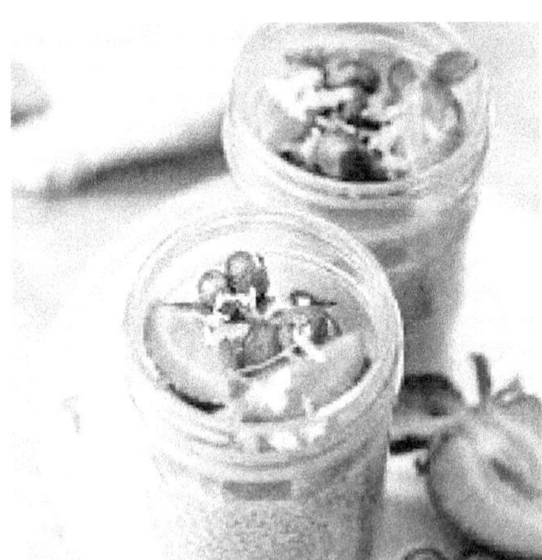

CHIA SEED PUDDING

Serves: 1
Calories: 379 per serving

Ingredients

- 2 tbsp chia seeds
- 1 ¼ cup non-dairy milk
- ½ tsp vanilla extract
- ½ tsp maple syrup

Directions

1. Mix together all the ingredients, cover. Put in refrigerator overnight.

2. By the morning the seeds will be hydrated and have the consistency of a pudding.

3. Pair with your favorite toppings. Fruit and oatmeal work well. Serve and enjoy!

LUNCH RECIPE

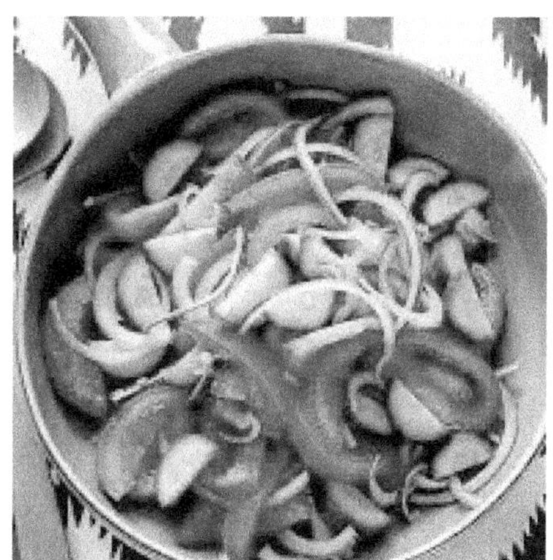

TOMATO, ONION, AND CUCUMBER SALAD

Serves: 4
Calories: 84 per serving

Ingredients

- 4 medium tomatoes, cut into wedges
- 2 medium cucumbers, sliced
- ½ large onion (of your choice), thinly sliced

- 3 tbsp Parsley, chopped
- pinch of salt and pepper
- 1 tbsp extra virgin olive oil
- 2 tsp balsamic vinegar

Directions

1. Prepare vegetables and parsley; wash, dry, and cut.
2. Put in a large bowl and gently toss to mix.
3. Add salt, pepper, oil, and vinegar and gently toss again.
4. Plate, serve, and enjoy!

DINNER RECIPE

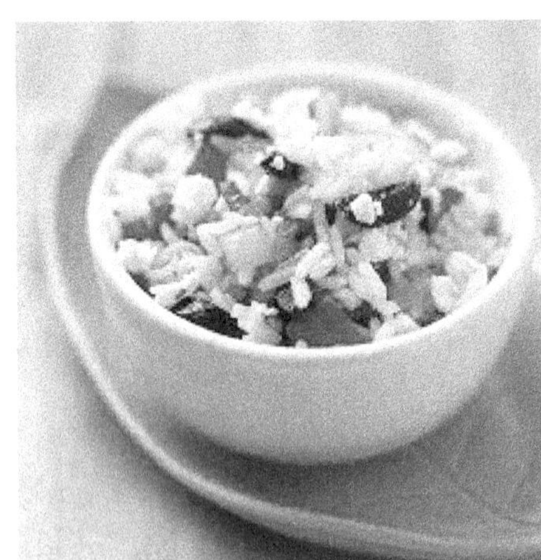

GREEK SALAD RICE

Serves: 6
Calories: 293 per serving

Ingredients

- 2 cups brown rice, cooked
- juice of 1/2 lemon
- 10 cherry tomatoes, halved
- 1/3 red onion, diced
- ½ cucumber, diced
- 2 tsp extra virgin olive oil
- 1 tsp balsamic vinegar
- 1 tsp dried oregano

Directions

1. Cook brown rice to package directions, mix in dried oregano. Set aside.

2. Prepare vegetables. Wash, dry, and cut tomatoes, and cucumbers. Cut the onion.

3. Add to a large bowl with cooled off rice, mix until combined.

4. Add olive oil, balsamic vinegar, and lemon juice over top. Just it one more toss.

5. Plate, serve, and enjoy!

Day 2

Shopping list

- Tofu
- Non-dairy milk
- Onion
- Jalapeno
- Tomatoes
- Cilantro
- Potato
- Tortilla wraps
- Chili powder
- Salt and pepper
- Lemon juice
- Lime juice
- Clove garlic
- Avocado
- Black beans
- Cumin
- Chili powder
- Garlic powder
- Portobello mushroom caps
- Red bell pepper
- Orange bell pepper
- Salt and pepper
- Virgin olive oil

BREAKFAST RECIPE

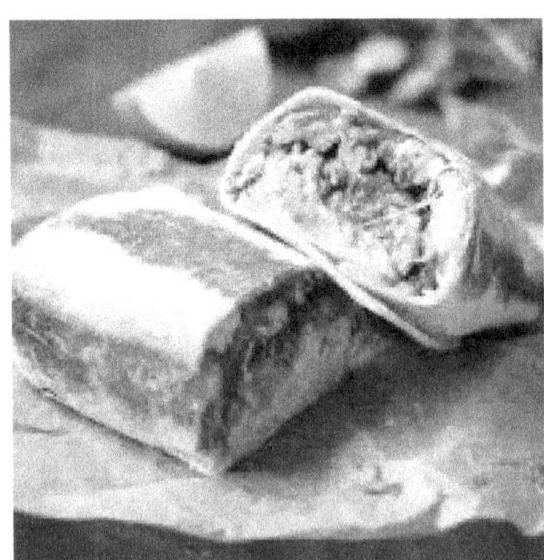

HEARTY BREAKFAST WRAP

Serves: 2
Calories: 310 per serving

Ingredients

- 1 cup extra firm tofu
- 2 tbsp plain unsweetened non-dairy milk of your choice
- ¼ onion, diced
- ¼ jalapeno, diced
- ½ tomato, diced
- ¼ cup cilantro, chopped
- 1 large potato

- 2 tortilla wraps
- 1 tsp chili powder
- 1 tsp onion powder
- pinch of salt and pepper
- 1 tsp lemon juice
- 1 tsp lime juice
- 1 clove garlic, minced

Directions

1. Prepare salsa. Wash, dry, and cut tomatoes, cilantro, and jalapeno. Cut onion and garlic. Juice lemon and lime. Combine vegetables with lemon juice, and lime juice. Mix together well and set aside.

2. Prepare potatoes. Wash, peel, and cut potatoes. The smaller you cut the potatoes the faster they will cook. Add to pan on medium heat, seasoning with a pinch of salt and pepper. Set aside.

3. Prepare tofu scramble. Drain, pat dry, and crumble extra firm tofu. Heat olive oil in the pan on medium heat. Add the crumbled tofu, chili powder, and onion powder. Add plant-based milk and cook for another minute or two until done.

4. Lay out tortillas. Spoon on the scramble, potatoes, and salsa. Wrap, serve, and enjoy!

LUNCH RECIPE

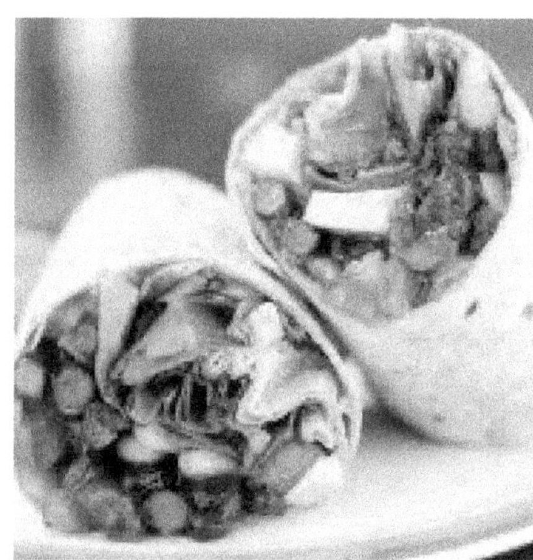

AVOCADO AND BLACK BEAN WRAP

Serves: 2
Calories: 450 per serving

Ingredients

- 1 avocado, sliced
- 2 tortilla wraps
- 1 can black beans
- 1 tomato, diced
- 1/2 tsp cumin
- ½ tsp chili powder
- ½ tsp garlic powder
- ½ tsp onion powder

Directions

1. Drain and rinse beans.

2. Warm skillet to medium heat and add beans, cumin, garlic powder, onion powder, and chili powder.

3. Stir frequently until beans are warmed through.

4. Cut avocado and tomatoes.

5. Allow beans to cool for a moment. Add to wraps. Place tomatoes and avocado on top. Wrap, serve, and enjoy!

DINNER RECIPE

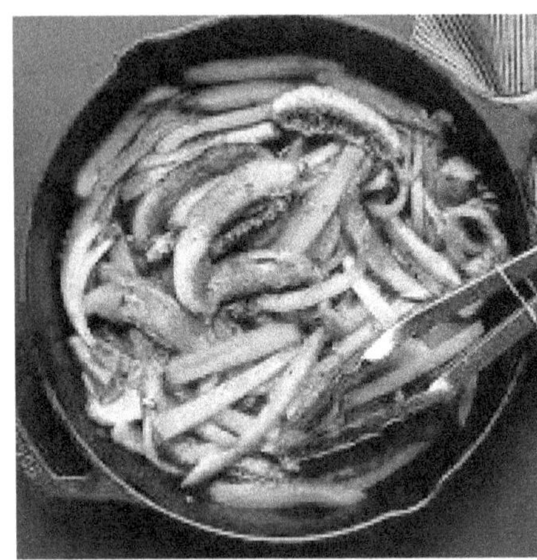

PORTOBELLO MUSHROOM FAJITAS

Serves: 2
Calories: 227 per serving

Ingredients

- 2 portobello mushroom caps, cut into thick slices (to your liking)
- 1 red bell pepper
- 1 orange bell pepper
- 1 medium onion
- Pinch of salt and pepper
- 1 tsp cumin
- 1/2 tsp garlic powder
- 1 tsp onion powder
- 1 tsp chili powder
- 2 tsp extra virgin olive oil
- Tortillas

Directions

1. Wash, dry, and cut vegetables.

2. Heat olive oil in a skillet. Add onions, mushrooms, peppers, salt, pepper, garlic powder, cumin, onion powder, and chili powder. Mix well until vegetables are all coated.

3. Cook until vegetables are warmed through and cooked to your liking.

4. Add to tortilla and top with any other toppings you like; avocado, tomatoes, salsa, guacamole, vegan cheese, or vegan sour cream.

Day 3

Shopping list

- Tofu
- Non-dairy milk
- Onion
- Jalapeno
- Tomatoes
- Cilantro
- Potato
- Tortilla wraps
- Chili powder
- Salt and pepper
- Lemon juice
- Lime juice
- Clove garlic
- Avocado
- Black beans
- Cumin
- Chili powder
- Garlic powder
- Portobello mushroom caps
- Red bell pepper
- Orange bell pepper
- Salt and pepper
- Virgin olive oil
- Spinach

BREAKFAST RECIPE

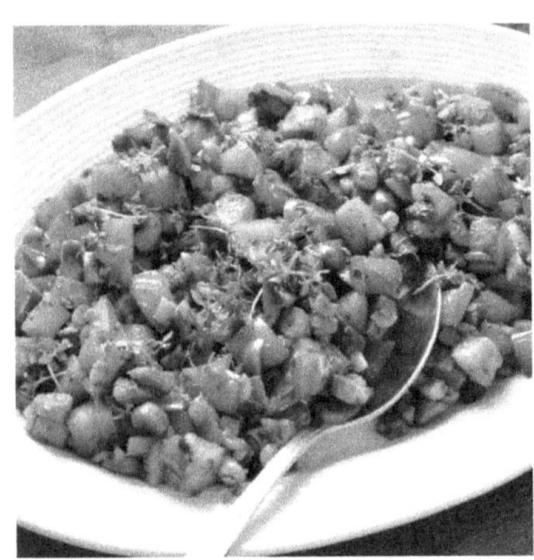

POTATO HASH

Serves: 2
Calories: 308 per serving

Ingredients

- 2 large potatoes, diced
- 1 medium onion, diced
- 1 tsp extra virgin olive oil
- 1 cup mushrooms
- 1 cup spinach
- Pinch of salt and pepper
- 1 tsp garlic powder
- 1 tsp onion powder
- 1 tsp chili powder

Directions

1. Prepare vegetables; wash and cut potatoes, onion, mushrooms. Wash spinach and set all aside.

2. Heat a skillet with olive oil at medium heat. Add potatoes, and cook, stirring occasionally until tender.

3. Add onions, mushrooms, salt, pepper, garlic powder, chili powder, and onion powder. Cook until onions are tender, stirring often.

4. Add spinach, cook until wilted to your liking.

5. Let cool for a couple of minutes. Plate, serve, and enjoy!

LUNCH RECIPE

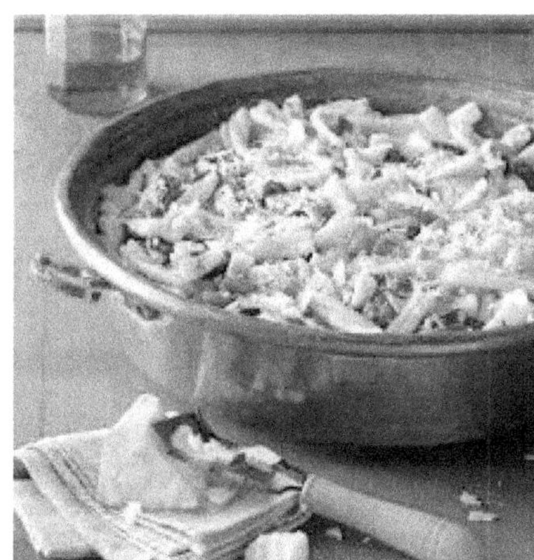

ONE POT BASIL AND VEGETABLE PASTA

Serves: 8
Calories: 196 per serving

Ingredients

- 1 lbs package of pasta of your choice
- 1 bunch basil, stems removed
- Pinch of salt and pepper
- 3 cloves of garlic, minced
- 1 red bell pepper, sliced
- 8 asparagus, cut into pieces
- 1 cup mushrooms, sliced
- 1 onion, diced
- 1 tbsp olive oil (roughly, may need more or less as per your liking)

Directions

1. Combine onion, garlic, basil, pepper, and asparagus and add water. Bring to a boil.
2. Cover pot and allow to boil for 10 minutes or until pasta is done.
3. Drain water. Add mushrooms to pasta and mix with the heat on medium.
4. Add olive oil, salt, and pepper. Toss to evenly coat all of the pasta and allow the mushrooms to warm through.
5. Plate, serve, and enjoy!

DINNER RECIPE

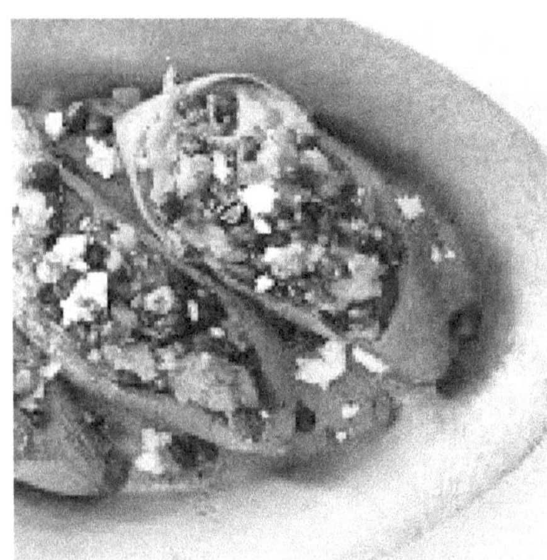

LOADED SWEET POTATOES

Serves: 2
Calories: 456 per serving

Ingredients

- 2 medium sweet potatoes
- 1 can black beans
- 1 tsp cumin
- 1 tsp garlic powder
- 1 tsp chili powder
- 1 tsp onion powder
- 1 medium tomato, diced
- 1/2 medium onion, diced
- 1 cup of corn

Directions

1. Preheat oven to 400 °F.

2. Prepare sweet potato. Wash, dry, pierce with fork and place on a baking sheet. Cooking for 40 minutes or until done.

3. In a skillet heat a small amount of olive oil over medium heat. Add black beans, corn, onion cumin, garlic powder, chili powder, and onion powder. Stirring frequently until thoroughly warmed through and onions go soft.

4. Prepare tomato; wash, dry, cut.

5. When sweet potatoes are finished. Cut them lengthwise and serve on a plate. Pour the bean mixture over the sweet potatoes. Plate, serve, and enjoy!

Day 4

Shopping list

- Tofu
- Non-dairy milk
- Onion
- Jalapeno
- Tomatoes
- Cilantro
- Potato
- Tortilla wraps
- Chili powder
- Salt and pepper
- Lemon juice
- Lime juice
- Clove garlic
- Avocado
- Black beans
- Cumin
- Chili powder
- Garlic powder
- Portobello mushroom caps
- Red bell pepper
- Orange bell pepper
- Salt and pepper
- Virgin olive oil
- Spinach
- Potatoes
- Spinach
- Parsley
- Carrots
- Vegetable broth

BREAKFAST RECIPE

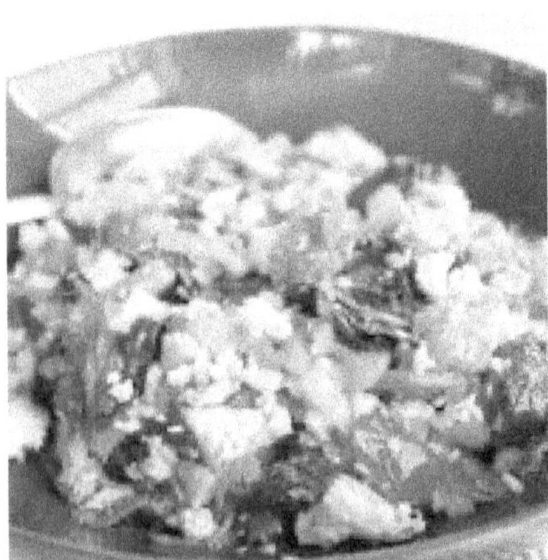

TOFU SCRAMBLE WITH VEGETABLES

Serves: 2
Calories: 300 per serving

Ingredients

- ¾ cup extra firm tofu
- pinch of salt and pepper
- garlic powder
- onion powder
- 1 tsp extra virgin olive oil

- ½ bell pepper (color of your choice), diced
- ¼ onion, diced
- 2 tbsp plain unsweetened non-dairy milk of your choice

Directions

1. Prepare vegetables. Wash and cut bell pepper. Cut onion, set all aside.

2. Prepare tofu; drain, pat dry, and crumble. Stir frequently for a few minutes

3. Heat olive oil in the pan on medium heat. Add the crumbled tofu, salt, pepper, garlic powder, onion powder. Add plant-based milk and cook for another minute or two until done.

4. Add onions and peppers to the scramble. Cook stirring frequently until the vegetables are softer, to your liking. Be careful to not overcook the tofu scramble. Alternatively, you can make them in a separate pan then combine and mix.

5. Serve with some toast or on a wrap for a full breakfast. Enjoy!

LUNCH RECIPE

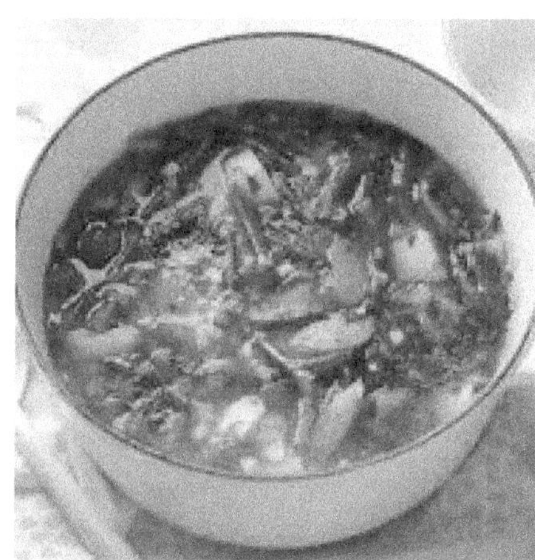

Vegetable Soup

Serves: 8
Calories: 139 per serving

Ingredients

- 2 tbsp extra virgin olive
- 4 stalks of celery, chopped
- 4 cloves of garlic, minced
- 1 onion, diced
- 2 tbsp tomato puree
- 2 tsp cumin
- 2 tsp onion powder
- 1 tsp chili powder
- 1 can stewed tomatoes
- 2 potatoes, diced
- 3 cups spinach
- 1 cup parsley, chopped
- 3 carrots, diced
- Pinch of salt and pepper
- 8 cups vegetable broth

Directions

1. Heat olive oil. Add onion, garlic, celery, and carrots. Cook until onions are tender. Stirring often.

2. Add tomato puree, salt, pepper, cumin, onion powder, and chili powder. Let cook for a couple of minutes.

3. Add potatoes, stewed tomatoes, and vegetable broth.

4. Boil for 10 minutes. Then bring down to a simmer for at 30 minutes or until potatoes are cooked through. The smaller the potatoes are cut, the faster they will cook.

5. Add spinach and parsley, stir well and frequently until spinach is wilted to your liking.

6. Let cool slightly, serve, and enjoy!

DINNER RECIPE

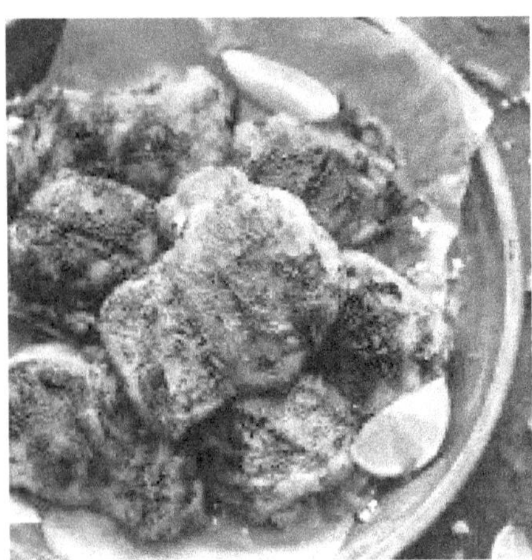

Grilled Cajun Pineapple and Lemon Rice

Serves: 4
Calories: 276 per serving

Ingredients

- 1 large pineapple, core and skin removed and cut into steaks
- Cajun seasoning (prepackaged or a mix of your own - chili powder, onion powder, garlic powder, a pinch of salt and pepper)

- 4 cups of brown rice, cooked
- juice of one lemon
- 3/4 cup cilantro, chopped

Directions

1. Cook rice to directions on the package but add the lemon juice to the water while cooking.

2. Chop cilantro, set aside.

3. When rice is finished, fluff with a fork and mix in cilantro.

4. Prepare pineapple, wash and remove the skin. Remove the core and cut into thick pieces. 8 pieces will be 1 serving for 4 people.

5. Mix in the cajun seasoning with olive oil and brush onto pineapple pieces.

6. Grill on medium heat for roughly 8 minutes and flip. Pineapple should still be juicy and tender but begin to brown around edges. Cook for another couple of minutes.

7. Plate the rice and pineapple, serve, and enjoy!

Day 5

Shopping list

- Tofu
- Non-dairy milk
- Onion
- Jalapeno
- Tomatoes
- Cilantro
- Potato
- Tortilla wraps
- Chili powder
- Salt and pepper
- Lemon juice
- Lime juice
- Clove garlic
- Avocado
- Black beans
- Cumin
- Chili powder
- Garlic powder
- Portobello mushroom caps
- Red bell pepper
- Orange bell pepper
- Salt and pepper
- Virgin olive oil
- Spinach
- Potatoes
- Spinach
- Parsley
- Carrots
- Vegetable broth

BREAKFAST RECIPE

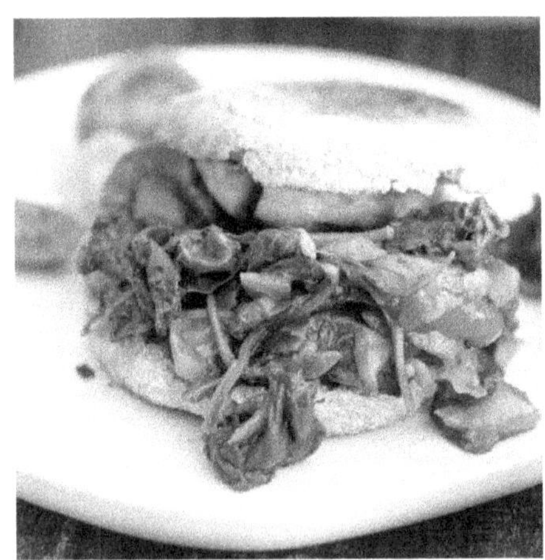

Mushroom English Muffin

Serves: 1
Calories: 194 per serving

Ingredients

- 3 cremini mushrooms, sliced
- 1 slice of red onion
- 1/4 cup spinach
- 1 slice of tomato
- Pinch of salt and pepper
- Pinch of red pepper flakes
- English muffin
- 1 tsp extra virgin olive oil

Directions

1. Clean dirt off of mushrooms with a damp paper towel and slice them.
2. Wash, dry, and cut tomato. Slice red onion. Wash spinach. Set all aside.
3. Warm olive oil over medium heat in a skillet. Place mushroom slices in skillet and season with salt, pepper, and red pepper flakes. Stirring frequently to cook.
4. Toast English muffin.
5. Place mushrooms, spinach, tomato, and onion on English muffin.
6. Plate, serve and enjoy!

LUNCH RECIPE

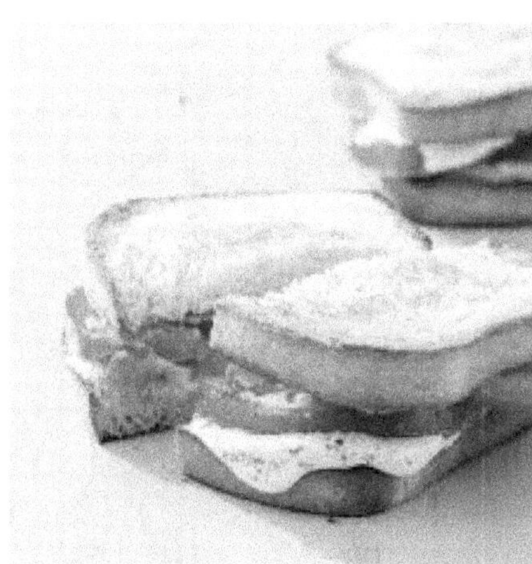

TOMATO SANDWICH

Serves: 1
Calories: 170 per serving

Ingredients

- ½ a large tomato
- pinch of salt and pepper
- 1 tbsp hummus
- 2 slices of whole grain bread

Directions

1. Wash, dry, and cut tomatoes. Slice to your preferred thickness.
2. Toast bread to your liking.
3. Spoon hummus over one side, add tomato on top, sprinkle salt and pepper to your liking.
4. Cut in half, serve and enjoy!

DINNER RECIPE

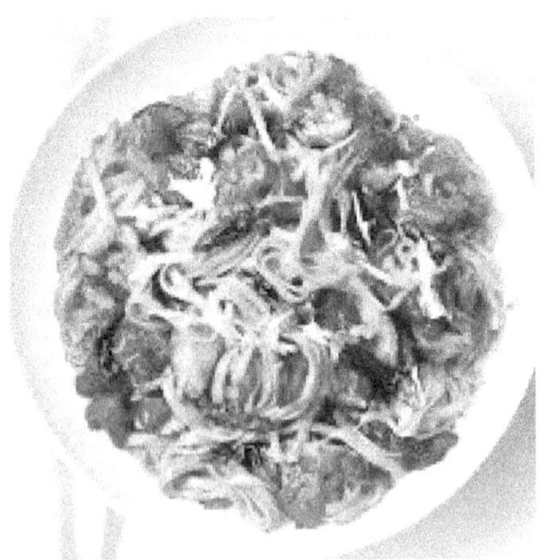

ROASTED VEGETABLE PASTA

Serves: 3
Calories: 353 per serving

Ingredients

- Package of pasta, roughly 6 oz
- 1 large zucchini
- 1 medium red onion
- 1 cup of corn
- 1 bell pepper
- Extra virgin olive oil
- ½ cup of basil, chopped

Directions

1. Preheat oven to 375 °F.
2. Prepare vegetables; wash, dry, cut, and place on the baking sheet. Bake until done, roughly 45 minutes.
3. While vegetables are roasting to cook the pasta. Cook for roughly 10 minutes or until pasta is done.
4. Drain the pasta and put back into the large pot.
5. When vegetables are cooked, take them out of the oven and add them to the large pot.
6. Add a drizzle of olive oil, salt, pepper, and basil. Toss until well combined.
7. Plate, serve, and enjoy!

Day 6

Shopping list

- Tofu
- Non-dairy milk
- Onion
- Jalapeno
- Tomatoes
- Cilantro
- Potato
- Tortilla wraps
- Chili powder
- Salt and pepper
- Lemon juice
- Lime juice
- Clove garlic
- Avocado
- Black beans
- Cumin
- Chili powder
- Garlic powder
- Portobello mushroom caps
- Red bell pepper
- Orange bell pepper
- Salt and pepper
- Virgin olive oil
- Spinach
- Potatoes
- Spinach
- Parsley
- Carrots
- Vegetable broth

BREAKFAST RECIPE

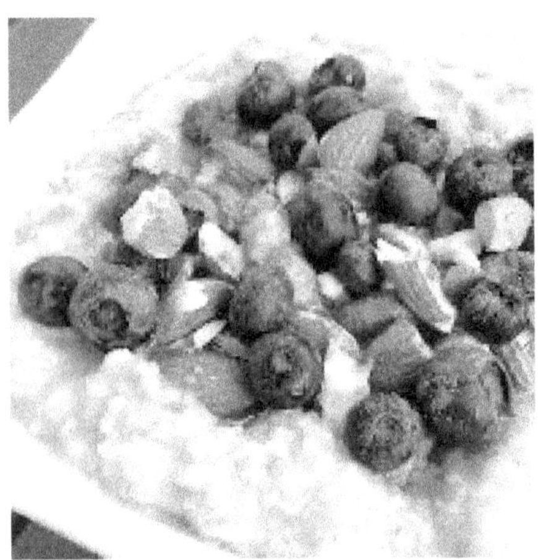

BERRY ALMOND STEEL CUT OATS

Serves: 1
Calories: 358 per serving

Ingredients

- 1 cup steel cut oats, cooked
- Splash of unsweetened vanilla almond milk
- 1/2 tsp cinnamon
- 1/4 cup strawberries, diced
- 1/4 cup blueberries
- 1/4 cup raspberries
- a drizzle of maple syrup

Directions

1. Cook steel cut oats to package directions. You're going to want about 1 cup of cooked oats for a serving.

2. Prepare fruit. Wash, dry, cut berries, set aside.

3. Put oats in a serving bowl, add a splash of almond milk, and a drizzle of maple syrup over top, both to your liking.

4. Sprinkle cinnamon on top with the berries. Serve and enjoy!

LUNCH RECIPE

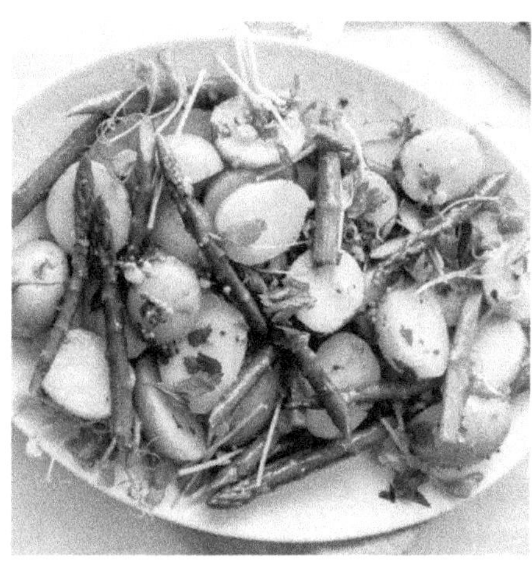

WARM POTATO SALAD

Serves: 4
Calories: 191 per serving

Ingredients

- 4 potatoes, diced
- 1 cup green onions, sliced
- 1 tbsp extra virgin olive oil
- Pinch of salt and pepper
- 8 asparagus, cut into pieces
- balsamic vinegar

Directions

1. Wash, dry, and cut potatoes.
2. Boil in salted water.
3. Prepare asparagus and green onion, wash, dry, cut.
4. Heat olive oil. Add asparagus and stir frequently until cooked to your liking.
5. When done add to the bowl of potatoes and add the green onion.
6. Add a drizzle of extra virgin olive oil and balsamic vinegar, gently toss until combined.
7. Plate and serve warm. Enjoy!

DINNER RECIPE

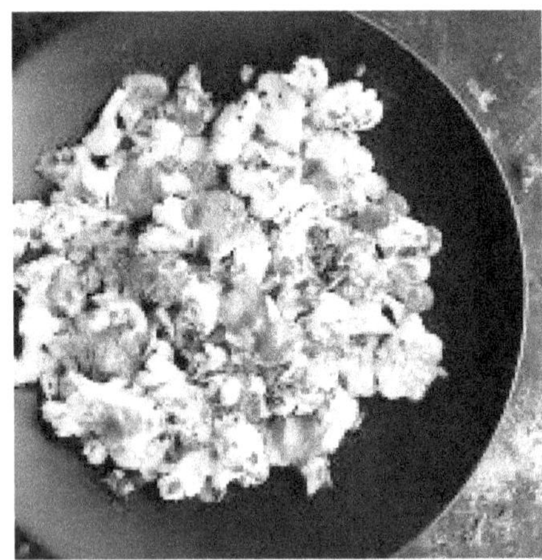

Roasted Cauliflower with Chimichurri Sauce

Serves: 2
Calories: 299 per serving

Ingredients

- 1 large head of cauliflower
- 3 tbsp extra virgin olive oil
- 1/3 cup cilantro, chopped
- 1/3 cup parsley, chopped
- 2 tbsp red wine vinegar
- 1 jalapeno, seeds removed, finely chopped
- 2 cloves of garlic, minced
- pinch of salt and pepper

Directions

1. Preheat oven to 425°F.

2. Wash, dry, and cut cauliflower. Put in a bowl. Toss with roughly 2 tbsp oil, salt, and pepper. You want just enough oil to coat the cauliflower lightly and evenly. Add little bits at a time to not over add.

3. Put cauliflower on a baking sheet. Bake for 20 minutes, flip, and bake another 5 minutes or until done.

4. Make the sauce by mixing the cilantro, 2 tbsp oil, parsley, garlic, vinegar, jalapeno, and a small pinch of salt.

5. When cauliflower is done, plate and pour the sauce over them. Serve and enjoy!

Day 7

Shopping list

- Tofu
- Non-dairy milk
- Onion
- Jalapeno
- Tomatoes
- Cilantro
- Potato
- Tortilla wraps
- Chili powder
- Salt and pepper
- Lemon juice
- Lime juice
- Clove garlic
- Avocado
- Black beans
- Cumin
- Chili powder
- Garlic powder
- Portobello mushroom caps
- Red bell pepper
- Orange bell pepper
- Salt and pepper
- Virgin olive oil
- Spinach
- Potatoes
- Spinach
- Parsley
- Carrots
- Vegetable broth

BREAKFAST RECIPE

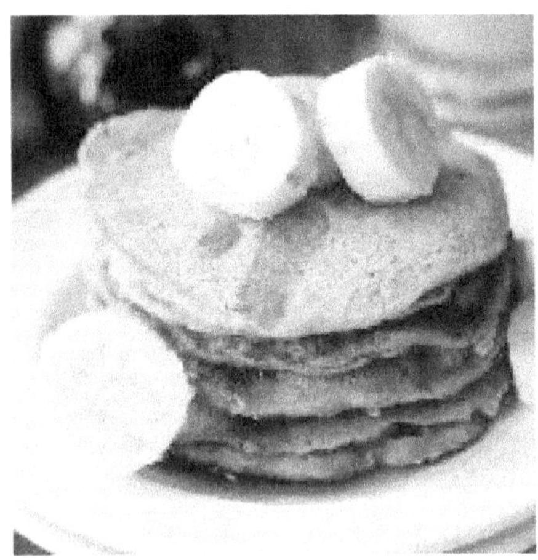

Banana Pumpkin Pie Pancakes

Serves: 4
Calories: 345 per serving

Ingredients

- 3 cups oat flour
- 1 1/2 tsp pumpkin pie spice
- 2 cups unsweetened vanilla almond milk
- 2 overripe bananas

Directions

1. Mash bananas in a large bowl

2. Add flour, pumpkin pie spice, and almond milk. Use a hand mixer and mix until batter forms.

3. Heat non-stick skillet on medium.

4. Pour batter in equal parts into the skillet. You can use a measuring cup to ensure size consistency. 1/3 cup measuring cup works best.

5. Once bubbles begin to form over the top of the pancakes and the edges are set, flip the cake and cook until golden.

6. Plate and top with some more bananas, a drizzle of maple syrup, or whatever you prefer. Serve and enjoy!

LUNCH RECIPE

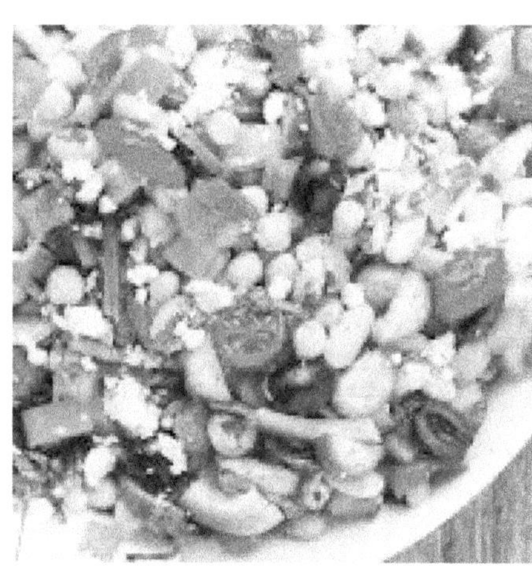

BEAN SALAD

Serves: 4
Calories: 200 per serving

Ingredients

- 1 can mixed beans
- ½ large red onion, diced
- 4 stalks of celery

- 1 large tomato, diced and seeds removed
- ½ large English cucumber, diced
- 2 large carrots, shredded

Directions

1. Drain and rinse beans, add them to a large bowl.
2. Cut onion add to bowl.
3. Wash, dry, and cut the celery, tomatoes, and cucumber. Wash, dry, and shred the carrots. Add all to bowl.
4. Add dressing, toss gently until mixed well.
5. Serve and enjoy!

DINNER RECIPE

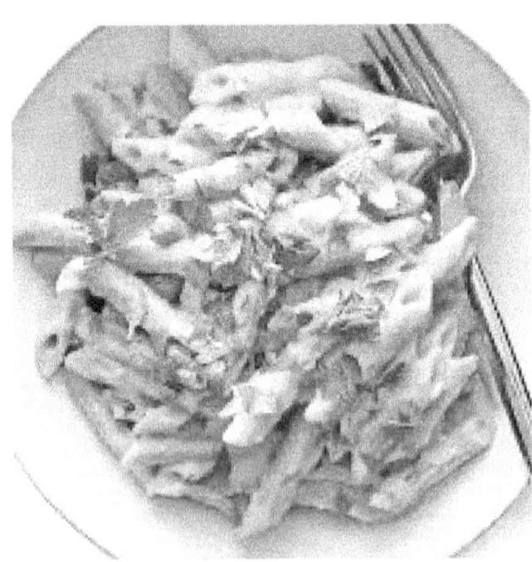

Chickpea Pasta

Serves: 3
Calories: 496 per serving

Ingredients

- ½ onion, diced
- 1 package chickpea pasta
- 3 cloves garlic, minced
- 1 zucchini, diced
- 2 carrots, diced
- 1 eggplant, diced
- 1 large can chopped tomatoes (about 400 g)
- ½ cup basil, chopped
- 1 can tomato or pasta sauce

Directions

1. Cook chickpea pasta to directions. Drain.
2. Heat olive oil in a skillet over medium heat. Add onions, garlic, zucchini, eggplant, and carrots. Allow them to cook while frequently stirring.
3. Add tomatoes, tomato sauce, basil, and pasta.
4. Stir and heat through.
5. Plate, serve, and enjoy!

Day 8

Shopping list

- Tofu
- Non-dairy milk
- Onion
- Jalapeno
- Tomatoes
- Cilantro
- Potato
- Tortilla wraps
- Chili powder
- Salt and pepper
- Lemon juice
- Lime juice
- Clove garlic
- Avocado
- Black beans
- Cumin
- Chili powder
- Garlic powder
- Portobello mushroom caps
- Red bell pepper
- Orange bell pepper
- Salt and pepper
- Virgin olive oil
- Spinach
- Potatoes
- Spinach
- Parsley
- Carrots
- Vegetable broth

BREAKFAST RECIPE

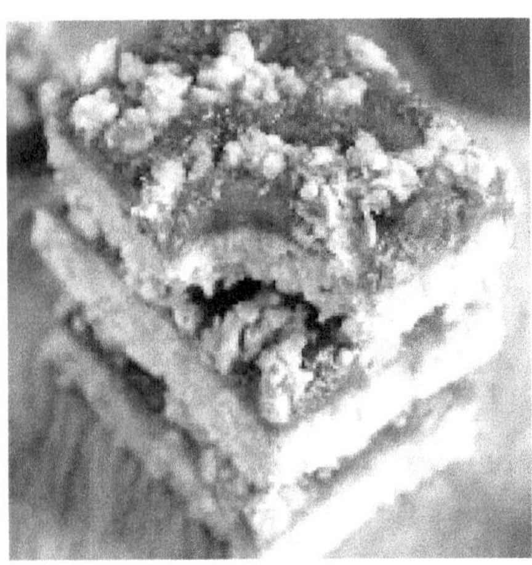

Banana Strawberry Bars

Serves: 12
Calories: 165 per serving

Ingredients

- 2 ripe bananas
- 1 ½ cups dates, pitted
- 3 cups rolled oats
- ½ tsp cinnamon
- ½ tsp nutmeg
- 1/4 tsp cardamom
- 1 ½ tbsp baking powder
- 1 1/2 tsp vanilla extract
- 1 cup strawberries, diced

Directions

1. Preheat the oven to 375 °F.
2. Line a 9x9 inch baking pan with parchment paper, placing paper over the sides as well.
3. In a bowl mix half of the oats, vanilla, nutmeg, cinnamon, cardamom, and baking powder together. Set aside.
4. In a blender blend together the rest of the oats, bananas, a splash of vanilla, and the apple juice (without the dates) until smooth
5. Add dates and blend for a moment until they are to your liking.
6. Add the strawberries into the mixture and pour it onto the baking pan.
7. Bake for roughly 30-40 minutes until cooked through.
8. Allow to cool and cut into 12. Serve and enjoy!

LUNCH RECIPE

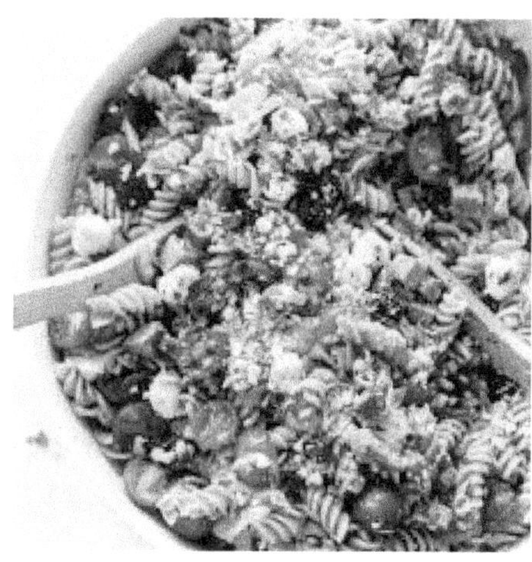

Pasta Salad

Serves: 6
Calories: 400 per serving

Ingredients

- 1 package of pasta
- 1 head of broccoli, chopped
- ½ red onion, diced
- 1 bell pepper, diced
- ½ can of black olives, halved
- 4 tbsp zesty Italian dressing

Directions

1. Cook pasta, drain. Add a splash of dressing and mix to stop the pasta from sticking together. Set aside in a large bowl in the refrigerator. Let cool completely.
2. Wash, dry, and cut broccoli and bell pepper. Add to pasta.
3. Cut onion and olives and add to pasta.
4. Pour in dressing and mix a little bit at a time, to your liking.
5. Serve and enjoy!

DINNER RECIPE

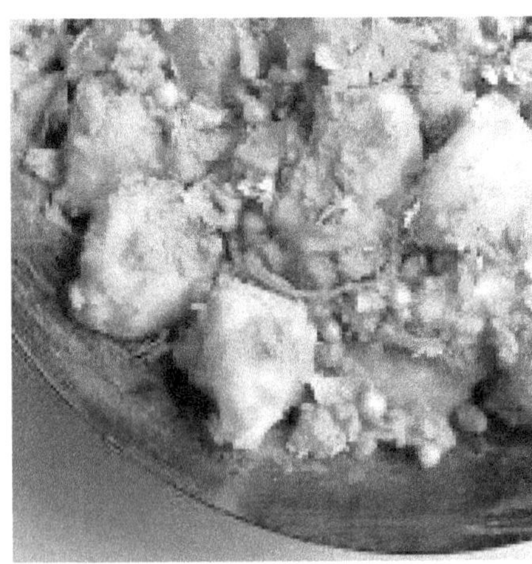

POTATO AND PEA CURRY

Serves: 4
Calories: 320 Per Serving

Ingredients

- 3 large potatoes
- 3 cloves garlic, minced
- 1 tbsp cumin
- 1 tbsp chili powder
- 1 cup coriander, chopped
- pinch of salt and pepper
- 3 tbsp vegetable oil
- 2 cups of water
- 1/2 onion, diced
- 1 cup of peas

Directions

1. Prepare potatoes; wash, peel, dry, and cut into small cubes.

2. Cook, stirring frequently for a minute.

3. Add potatoes, cook for a few minutes.

4. Add in cumin, chili, salt, and pepper. Stirring well. Add water, potatoes should be almost covered by the water. Add peas, frozen works best.

5. Potatoes should be cooked all the way through, check to see if they are cooked. If not after 20 minutes you may add another cup of water and cook again.

6. When the curry is done, and the right consistency and the potatoes are fully cooked add in the coriander and cook for a couple of minutes.

7. Plate, serve with rice or bread, and enjoy!

Day 9

Shopping list

- Tofu
- Non-dairy milk
- Onion
- Jalapeno
- Tomatoes
- Cilantro
- Potato
- Tortilla wraps
- Chili powder
- Salt and pepper
- Lemon juice
- Lime juice
- Clove garlic
- Avocado
- Black beans
- Cumin
- Chili powder
- Garlic powder
- Portobello mushroom caps
- Red bell pepper
- Orange bell pepper
- Salt and pepper
- Virgin olive oil
- Spinach
- Potatoes
- Spinach
- Parsley
- Carrots
- Vegetable broth

BREAKFAST RECIPE

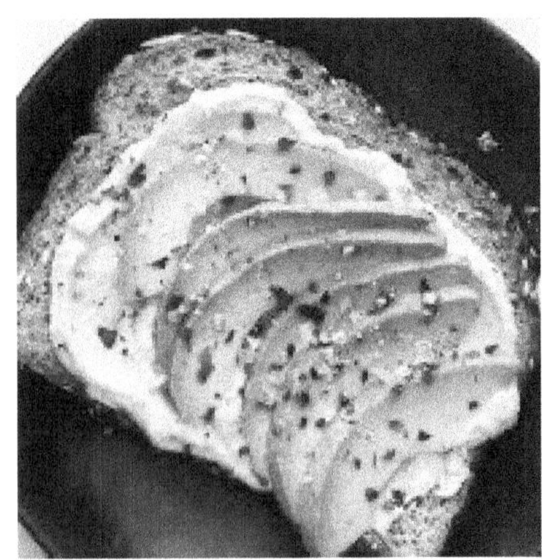

HUMMUS AND AVOCADO TOAST

Serves: 2
Calories: 247 per serving

Ingredients

- 2 pieces of whole grain bread
- 1 tbsp hummus
- ½ half an avocado, cut into slices
- ½ a tomato, cut into slices
- pinch of salt and pepper

Directions

1. Prepare vegetables; wash, dry, and cut tomato and avocado.

2. Toast bread to your liking.

3. Spread hummus over each slice of bread, place slices of tomato over the hummus and add a pinch of salt and pepper.

4. Top each piece of bread with avocado. Serve and enjoy!

LUNCH RECIPE

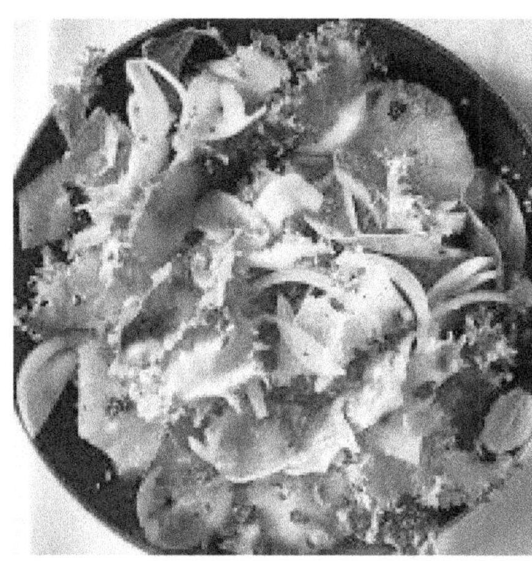

CITRUS SALAD

Serves: 4
Calories: 301 per serving

Ingredients

- 4 cups spinach
- ½ small red onion, diced
- 1 medium mandarin orange
- ½ a grapefruit
- 1 tbsp lemon juice
- 1 can chickpeas

Directions

1. Wash spinach, place in a large bowl.
2. Cut onion, peel orange and grapefruit, cut segments in half and add to spinach bowl.
3. Drain and rinse chickpeas.
4. Add lemon juice and toss gently.
5. Plate, serve, and enjoy!

DINNER RECIPE

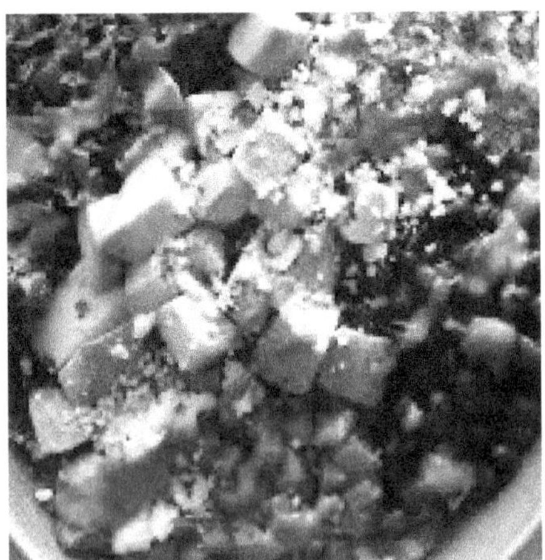

Sweet Potato Southwest Bowl

Serves: 3
Calories: 317 per serving

Ingredients

- 1 sweet potato, cut into cubes
- 1 cup brown rice, cooked
- 1/3 cup cilantro, chopped
- 1 cup corn, cooked but not warm
- 1/3 medium onion, chopped
- 1/3 jalapeno, chopped, seeds removed
- 1/3 large tomato, chopped, seeds removed
- 1 tsp cumin
- 1/2 tsp garlic powder
- 1 tsp onion powder
- 1 tsp chili powder
- extra virgin olive oil

Directions

1. Preheat oven to 375 °F.
2. Wash, peel, cut sweet potatoes. Place on a baking sheet in single layer and bake 30 minutes or until done.
3. While sweet potatoes are cooking, cook rice to directions on the package.
4. Heat a little olive oil, roughly a tsp just to coat the bottom, on medium heat in a skillet. Drain and rinse.
5. Add cumin, garlic powder, onion powder, chili powder, salt, and pepper to taste. Stirring frequently until beans are coated and warmed all the way through.
6. Wash, dry, and cut tomatoes, cilantro, and jalapenos. Mix in a small bowl with onion and corn.
7. Place rice in a bowl, add sweet potato on top, beans next to them, and corn salsa beside them both.
8. Serve and enjoy!

Day 10

Shopping list

- Tofu
- Non-dairy milk
- Onion
- Jalapeno
- Tomatoes
- Cilantro
- Potato
- Tortilla wraps
- Chili powder
- Salt and pepper
- Lemon juice
- Lime juice
- Clove garlic
- Avocado
- Black beans
- Cumin
- Chili powder
- Garlic powder
- Portobello mushroom caps
- Red bell pepper
- Orange bell pepper
- Salt and pepper
- Virgin olive oil
- Spinach
- Potatoes
- Spinach
- Parsley
- Carrots
- Vegetable broth

BREAKFAST RECIPE

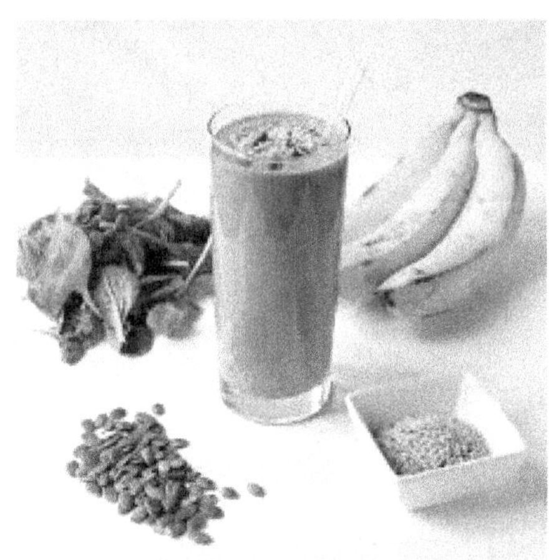

POWER BREAKFAST SMOOTHIE

Serves: 1
Calories: 377 per serving

Ingredients

- 1 1/2 cups spinach
- 1 banana
- 1 small apple
- 1 cup of orange juice
- 1 tsp ginger root, minced
- 1 tbsp chia seeds

Directions

1. Prepare ingredients; wash and cut apple, peel a banana, wash spinach, and mince ginger. Place them all into your blender.

2. Add orange juice and chia seeds

3. Blend until smooth. Serve and enjoy!

LUNCH RECIPE

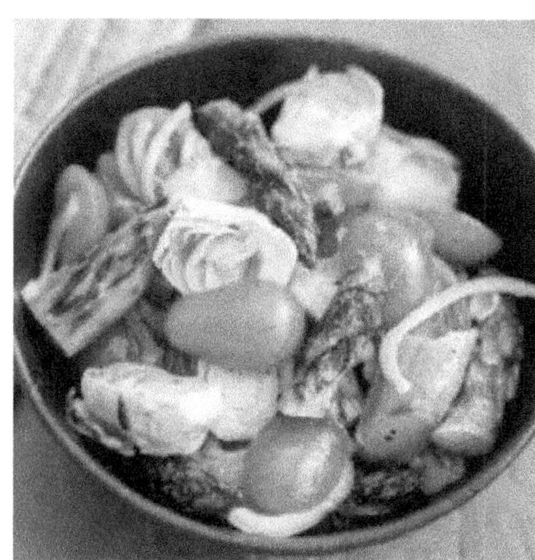

Asparagus and Artichoke Salad

Serves: 8
Prep time: 1 hour and 5 minutes

Ingredients

- 20 tender, fresh green asparagus stalks (woody stem removed, rinsed)
- 8 fresh, medium artichokes
- 4 tablespoons extra virgin olive oil
- 2 cloves garlic, peeled and chopped
- 1 ounce chopped pistachio nuts
- 1 large egg white
- 4 teaspoons chopped green onions + 1 green onion for garnish, chopped
- Juice of 1 lemon
- Salt and white pepper to taste

Directions

1. Fill a large pot ¾ of the way with water; add half the lemon juice and a generous sprinkle of salt.

2. Trim the artichokes by removing the leaves until you get to the light-yellow leaves. Set the hearts aside.

3. Place the artichoke leaves in boiling water. Cook 45 minutes. Once boiled, rinse under cold water.

4. Place the artichoke leaves in a food processor. Add the remaining lemon juice, half a glass of water (4 ounces), pinch of salt and pepper, pistachios, green onions, garlic, and egg white. Blend for 1 minute. Add the olive oil slowly. Continue to blend until smooth.

5. Cut up the artichoke hearts and arrange on plate. Place the asparagus over top. Drizzle the sauce over the artichokes and asparagus. Garnish with fresh green onions. Serve.

Nutritional Value (Amount per Serving)

Protein   5.9 g
Carbs: 11 g
Fat: 7 g

DINNER RECIPE

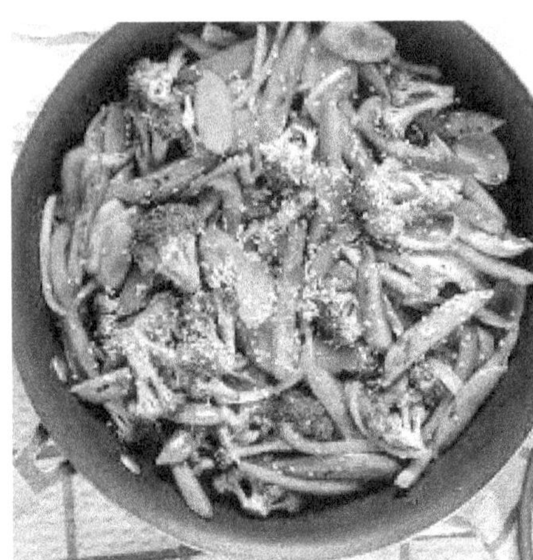

VEGETABLE STIR FRY

Serves: 4
Calories: 428 per serving

Another great classic that even the kids will be asking for seconds. Stir fry is cheap, easy, fast, and easily changed up how you like. Perfect for lunch or dinner.

Ingredients

- 2 cups brown rice, cooked
- 1 cup mushrooms, sliced
- 1 cup snap peas
- 1 medium onion, chopped
- 1 bell pepper

- 1 tbsp soy sauce
- 2 tsp cooking oil of your choice
- 1/3 cup water chestnuts, sliced
- 1 tbsp grated ginger

Directions

1. Cook brown rice, set aside
2. Prepare vegetables; wash, dry, cut. Grate ginger and set aside.

Day 11

Shopping list

- Tofu
- Non-dairy milk
- Onion
- Jalapeno
- Tomatoes
- Cilantro
- Potato
- Tortilla wraps
- Chili powder
- Salt and pepper
- Lemon juice
- Lime juice
- Clove garlic
- Avocado
- Black beans
- Cumin
- Chili powder
- Garlic powder
- Portobello mushroom caps
- Red bell pepper
- Orange bell pepper
- Salt and pepper
- Virgin olive oil
- Spinach
- Potatoes
- Spinach
- Parsley
- Carrots
- Vegetable broth

BREAKFAST RECIPE

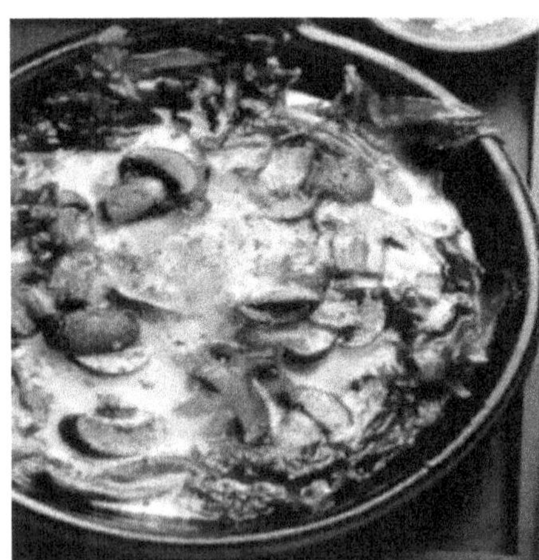

BAKED EGGS WITH SPINACH AND MUSHROOMS

Serves: 3
Prep time: 20 minutes

Ingredients

- 4 large eggs
- 3 cups chopped spinach
- 3 cups sliced mushrooms
- 1 green bell pepper, coarsely chopped
- 2 tablespoons extra virgin olive oil
- Salt and pepper to taste

Directions

1. Preheat oven to 400   F. Grease an 8x8 baking dish with olive oil.
2. Place the bell peppers, spinach, and mushrooms in the baking dish.
3. Carefully crack the eggs over the vegetables. Season with salt and pepper.
4. Bake until the whites are set, approximately 10 minutes.
5. Transfer to plates. Serve.

Nutritional Value (Amount per Serving)

Protein: 12.7 g
Carbs: 7.6 g
Fat: 9.9 g

LUNCH RECIPE

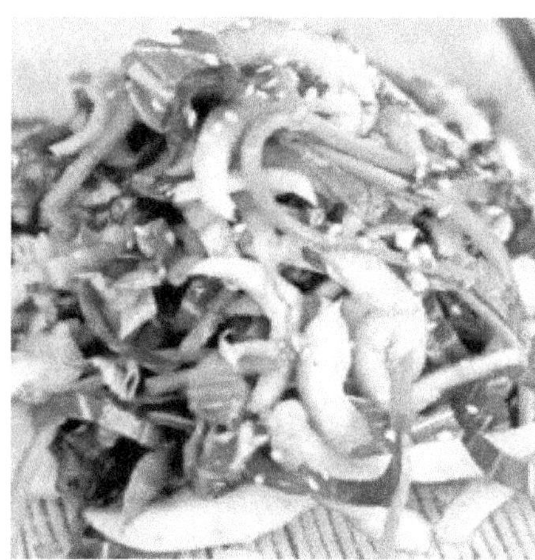

Pressure-Cooker Bok Choy Warm Salad

Serves: 3
Prep time: 10 minutes

Ingredients

- 1 bunch trimmed bok choy
- 2 cups water
- 2 tablespoons olive oil
- 2 tablespoons fresh-squeezed lime juice
- Salt and pepper to taste

Directions

1. Place the bok choy in the pressure cooker. Add enough water to cover.

2. Close lid. Set pressure to High. Cook 7 minutes.

3. Once cooked, allow the pressure to drop naturally, approximately 20 minutes.

4. Transfer to a serving platter. Drizzle lime juice and oil over. Sprinkle with salt and pepper. Serve.

Nutritional Value (Amount per Serving)

Protein: 8.5 g
Carbs: 9.9 g
Fat: 10.1 g

DINNER RECIPE

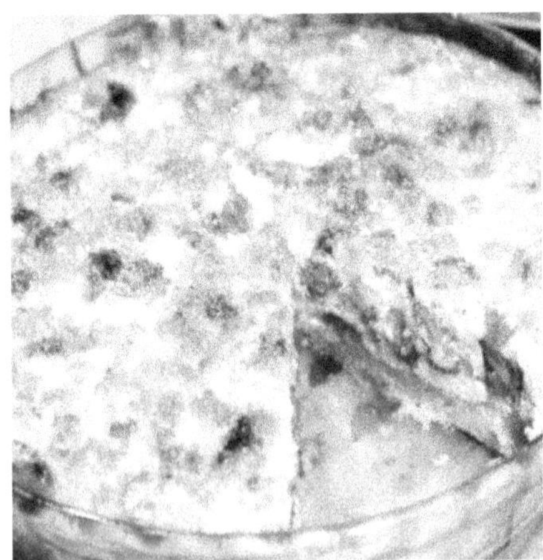

CRUSTLESS FETA MUSHROOM QUICHE

Serves: 6
Prep time: 45 minutes

Ingredients

- 8 ounces' button mushrooms, thinly sliced
- 1 clove garlic, minced
- 10 ounces thawed frozen spinach
- 4 large eggs
- 1 cup milk
- 2 ounces' feta cheese
- ¼ cup grated Parmesan
- ½ cup shredded mozzarella
- Salt & pepper to taste

Directions

1. Preheat oven to 400°F. Squeeze excess water out of the thawed spinach.

2. Heat a tablespoon or so of cooking oil in a large non-stick frying pan over medium heat.

3. Add the garlic and mushrooms. Sauté until tender, approximately 7 minutes.

4. Grease a large pie dish with non-stick spray. Arrange the spinach along the bottom of the pie dish. Pour the mushrooms and garlic over the spinach. Crumble feta cheese over top.

5. In a large bowl, whisk together the milk, eggs, and Parmesan cheese. Lightly season with pepper. Pour the egg mixture on top of the ingredients in the pie dish.

6. Sprinkle mozzarella over the top.

Nutritional Value (Amount per Serving)

Protein: 17 g
Carbs: 4 g
Fat: 18 g

Day 12

Shopping list

- Tofu
- Non-dairy milk
- Onion
- Jalapeno
- Tomatoes
- Cilantro
- Potato
- Tortilla wraps
- Chili powder
- Salt and pepper
- Lemon juice
- Lime juice
- Clove garlic
- Avocado
- Black beans
- Cumin
- Chili powder
- Garlic powder
- Portobello mushroom caps
- Red bell pepper
- Orange bell pepper
- Salt and pepper
- Virgin olive oil
- Spinach
- Potatoes
- Spinach
- Parsley
- Carrots
- Vegetable broth

BREAKFAST RECIPE

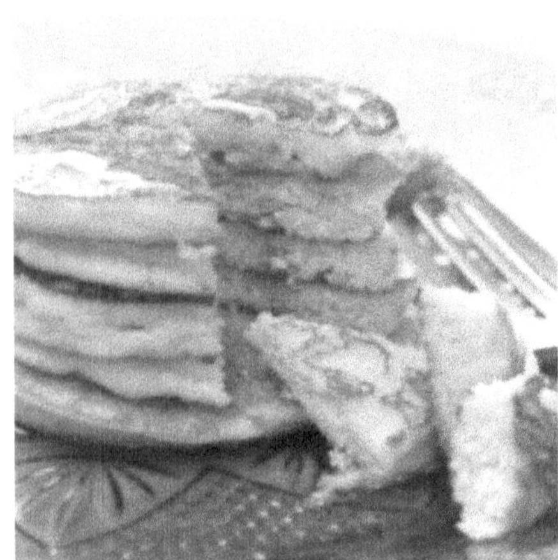

FLAXSEED COTTAGE PANCAKES

Serves: 6
Prep time: 15 minutes

Ingredients

- ½ cup ground flax seed meal
- 3 tablespoons cottage cheese
- 2 large eggs
- 2 tablespoons butter
- ½ cup heavy cream
- ¼ teaspoon gluten-free baking powder
- Coconut oil or olive oil for frying

Directions

1. Combine all the ingredients. Whisk together thoroughly.
2. Heat the oil.
3. Spoon ¾ cup of batter into the frying pan. Cook for 2 minutes per side.
4. Transfer onto plate. Serve with fresh berries or (keto-friendly) syrup.

Nutritional Value (Amount per Serving)

Protein: 6.1 g
Carbs: 4.5 g
Fat: 13 g

LUNCH RECIPE

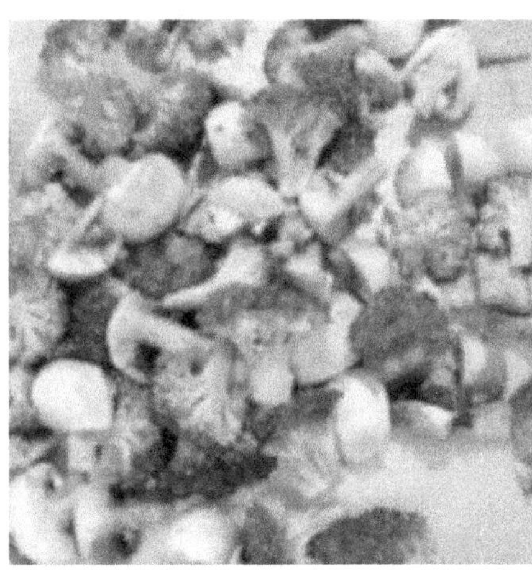

Mushroom & Broccoli Mix

Serves: 2
Prep time: 35 minutes

Ingredients

- 2 cups thinly sliced button mushrooms
- 4 cups broccoli
- 2 tablespoons minced garlic
- ½ teaspoon dried oregano
- 4 tablespoons grated Parmesan
- Salt and pepper to taste

Directions

1. The oven to be preheated to 400° F.
2. In a large bowl, combine mushrooms and broccoli. Add the olive oil and toss or stir to coat.
3. Season with salt, pepper, and oregano.
4. Transfer the broccoli and mushrooms to a baking dish. Bake 25 minutes.
5. Serve.

Nutritional Value (Amount per Serving)

Protein: 12.7 g
Carbs: 10.9 g
Fats: 3.5 g

DINNER RECIPE

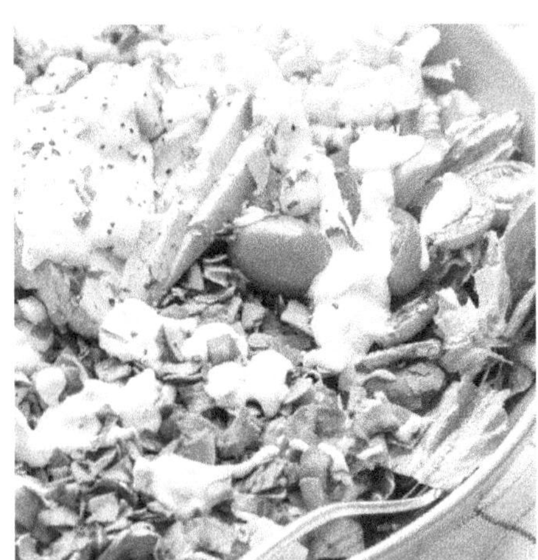

Easy and Healthy Spinach Cobb Salad

Serves: 2
Prep time: 10 minutes

Ingredients

- 2 boneless, skinless chicken breasts
- 4 slices bacon, cooked and crumbled
- 1 avocado, ripe and chopped
- 2 cups baby spinach, roughly chopped
- 1 cucumber, chopped
- 1 tomato, diced
- 2 hard-boiled eggs, chopped

Directions

1. Arrange the spinach on a serving platter.
2. Top the spinach with the remaining ingredients.
3. Serve and enjoy with ketogenic dressing.

Nutritional Value (Amount per Serving)

Protein: 31 g
Carbs: 6 g
Fat: 23 g

Day 13

Shopping list

- Tofu
- Non-dairy milk
- Onion
- Jalapeno
- Tomatoes
- Cilantro
- Potato
- Tortilla wraps
- Chili powder
- Salt and pepper
- Lemon juice
- Lime juice
- Clove garlic
- Avocado
- Black beans
- Cumin
- Chili powder
- Garlic powder
- Portobello mushroom caps
- Red bell pepper
- Orange bell pepper
- Salt and pepper
- Virgin olive oil
- Spinach
- Potatoes
- Spinach
- Parsley
- Carrots
- Vegetable broth

BREAKFAST RECIPE

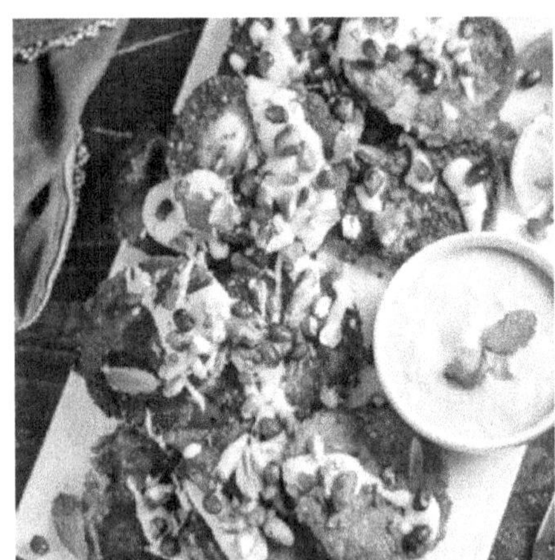

SUBTLE ROASTED EGGPLANT WITH FETA DIP

Serves: 12
Prep time: 40 minutes

Ingredients

- ¼ teaspoon cayenne pepper
- 2 tablespoons lemon juice
- 1 tablespoon finely chopped flat-leaf parsley
- ½ cup crumbled feta cheese
- 1 finely chopped small red bell pepper
- ¼ cup extra virgin olive oil

- 1 small chili pepper, seeded and minced
- 2 tablespoons chopped fresh basil
- 1 medium eggplant
- ¼ teaspoon salt
- Just a pinch of sugar

Directions

1. Preheat the broiler, positioning an oven rack about 6 inches below the heating element.
2. Line a baking pan with foil.
3. Gently poke holes all over the eggplant with a fork, and place on the pan.
4. Broil for about 18 minutes, turning the eggplant every 5 minutes.
5. Transfer the charred eggplant to a cutting board and let it cool.
6. In a medium-sized bowl, add the lemon juice.
7. Cut the eggplant in half lengthwise and scoop the flesh into the bowl.
8. Toss the flesh with the juice.
9. Add the oil and mash the mixture using a fork.
10. Stir in onion, feta, chili pepper, bell pepper, parsley, basil, salt and cayenne.
11. Mix well.
12. Season with sugar if desired.

Nutrition Value (Amount per Serving)

Protein: 2g
Carbs: 4g

Fats: 6g
Calories: 76

LUNCH RECIPE

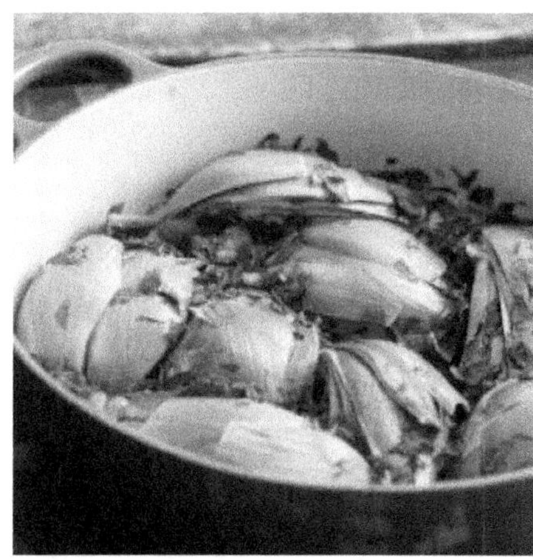

SLOW-COOKER SOUR BRAISED ARTICHOKES

Serves: 4
Prep time: 2-4 hours

Ingredients

- 4 artichokes
- 4 tablespoons lemon juice
- 2 tablespoons melted coconut butter
- Salt and pepper to taste
- Fresh chopped thyme

Directions

1. Rinse artichokes and trim by removing leaves, layer by layer, until light yellow leaves are left.
2. Place the artichokes, lemon juice, melted coconut butter and salt in the slow cooker.
3. Cook until the artichokes are fork tender.
4. Transfer to platter. Garnish with chopped thyme. Serve.

Nutritional Value (Amount per Serving)

Protein: 4.3 g
Carbs: 14.5 g
Fat: 5.6 g

DINNER RECIPE

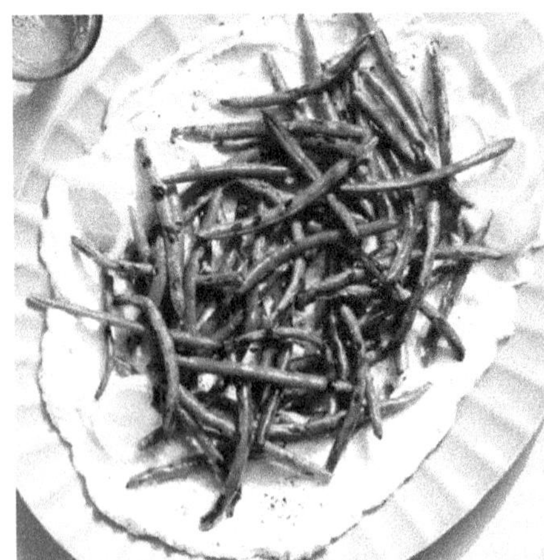

Lemon Green Beans & Caper Vinaigrette

Serves: 4
Prep time: 15 minutes

Ingredients

- 1 pound trimmed fresh green beans
- 3 tablespoons olive oil
- 2 tablespoons chopped capers
- Zest and juice from 1 lemon
- Salt and pepper to taste

Directions

1. Whisk together lemon juice, capers, oil, salt and pepper.
2. Boil and add 1 tablespoon of salt. Cook the green beans until tender, approximately 4-6 minutes.
3. Drain the beans and rinse in cold water.
4. Drizzle the caper vinaigrette over the beans and toss to coat. Transfer to plates. Serve.

Nutritional Value (Amount per Serving)

Protein: 1.8 g
Carbs: 8.7 g
Fat: 10.4 g

Day 14

Shopping list

- Tofu
- Non-dairy milk
- Onion
- Jalapeno
- Tomatoes
- Cilantro
- Potato
- Tortilla wraps
- Chili powder
- Salt and pepper
- Lemon juice
- Lime juice
- Clove garlic
- Avocado
- Black beans
- Cumin
- Chili powder
- Garlic powder
- Portobello mushroom caps
- Red bell pepper
- Orange bell pepper
- Salt and pepper
- Virgin olive oil
- Spinach
- Potatoes
- Spinach
- Parsley
- Carrots
- Vegetable broth

BREAKFAST RECIPE

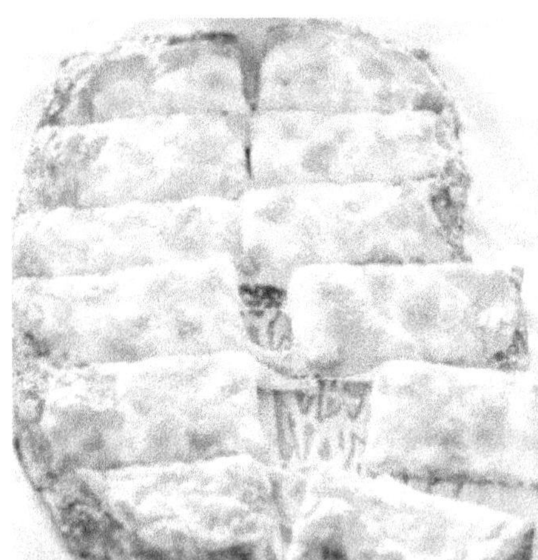

CAULIFLOWER MOZZARELLA STICKS

Serves: 6
Prep time: 50 minutes

Ingredients

- 1 medium cauliflower (to make 4 cups of cauliflower rice)
- 2 cups + 1 cup of mozzarella cheese
- 4 large eggs

- 4 cloves minced garlic
- 3 teaspoons fresh oregano
- Salt and pepper to taste
- Marinara sauce (for serving)

Directions

1. Preheat oven to 400 F.

2. Rinse the cauliflower and pat dry. Cut into florets.

3. Place the florets in a food processor. Pulse until rice-like consistency.

4. Transfer the cauliflower rice to microwavable container. Cover and microwave 10 minutes.

5. Pour the cauliflower rice. Add 2 cups of mozzarella cheese, eggs, oregano, salt, pepper and garlic. Stir together.

6. Line two large baking trays with parchment paper. Spread the mixture in a single, even layer on the baking trays. Bake 25 minutes, until golden brown.

7. Remove the trays from the oven. Return to oven until cheese melts.

8. Remove from oven. Let rest 5 minutes. Slice into sticks.

9. Place marinara sauce in a small bowl for dipping. Serve.

Nutritional Value (Amount per Serving)

Protein: 21.7 g
Carbs: 6.7 g
Fat: 13.9 g

LUNCH RECIPE

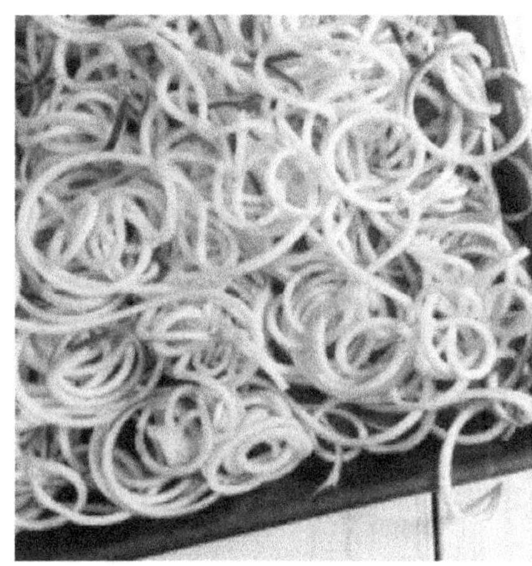

BASIL ZUCCHINI NOODLES

Serves: 3
Prep time: 15 minutes

Ingredients

- 3 tablespoons chopped fresh basil
- 2 cups zucchini noodles
- 4 tablespoons extra virgin olive oil
- 4 cloves garlic, mashed
- 1 teaspoon red pepper flakes
- ½ bell red pepper, chopped
- Salt and pepper to taste

Directions

1. Turn zucchini into noodles.
2. Heat olive oil. Add garlic, red pepper flakes and red pepper.
3. Add zucchini noodles. Stir well. Cook 3 minutes.
4. Transfer the zucchini noodle mixture to a plate. Garnish with basil. Serve.

Nutritional Value (Amount per Serving)

Protein: 3.9 g
Carbs: 5.6 g
Fat: 15.6 g

DINNER RECIPE

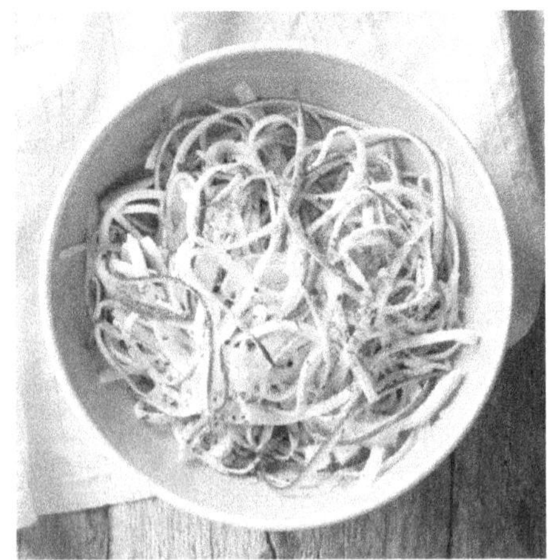

Ravishing Courgette Ribbon Salad

Serves: 4
Prep time: 15 minutes

Ingredients

- Juice of 1 lemon
- 2 tablespoons olive oil
- ½ a small package of chives, chopped
- ½ a small package of mint, chopped
- 300g courgettes
- Salt and pepper to taste

Directions

1. Add lemon juice, salt and pepper.
2. Whisk in olive oil and add the chopped herbs.
3. Pass the courgette through a spiralizer, making sure that the noodle attachment is placed so as to cut the courgette into spaghetti shape.
4. Tip the courgette ribbons into bowl.
5. Add dressing and toss well.
6. Serve!

Nutrition Value (Amount per Serving)

Protein: 29 g
Carbs: 65 g
Fats: 8 g

Day 15

Shopping list

- Tofu
- Non-dairy milk
- Onion
- Jalapeno
- Tomatoes
- Cilantro
- Potato
- Tortilla wraps
- Chili powder
- Salt and pepper
- Lemon juice
- Lime juice
- Clove garlic
- Avocado
- Black beans
- Cumin
- Chili powder
- Garlic powder
- Portobello mushroom caps
- Red bell pepper
- Orange bell pepper
- Salt and pepper
- Virgin olive oil
- Spinach
- Potatoes
- Spinach
- Parsley
- Carrots
- Vegetable broth

BREAKFAST RECIPE

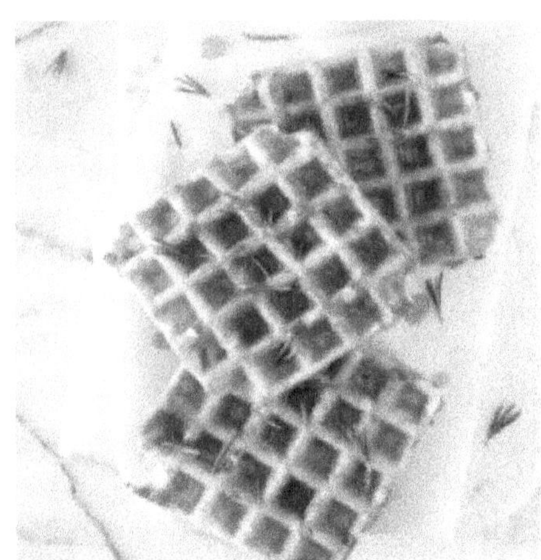

FLAXSEED SAVOURY WAFFLES

Serves: 6
Prep time: 15 minutes

Ingredients

- 5 large eggs
- 2 cups ground flaxseed
- 1 tablespoon baking powder (gluten-free)
- ½ teaspoon sea salt
- 1 cup water
- ½ cup melted coconut oil
- 1 tablespoon fresh herbs (sage, cilantro, parsley, basil)

Directions

1. Pre-heat waffle maker to medium heat.

2. Combine baking powder, salt, and flaxseed. Whisk thoroughly.

3. In a separate bowl, add eggs, oil and water. Using a whisk or handheld mixer, blend until fully combined. Pour the egg mixture in with the flaxseed mixture. Stir together. Let rest 5 minutes. Add the fresh herbs. Stir well.

4. Pour ¼ cup of mixture onto waffle maker. Cook 3 – 5 minutes.

5. Serve.

Nutritional Value (Amount per Serving)

Protein: 5.2 g
Carbs: 1.5 g
Fats: 16 g

LUNCH RECIPE

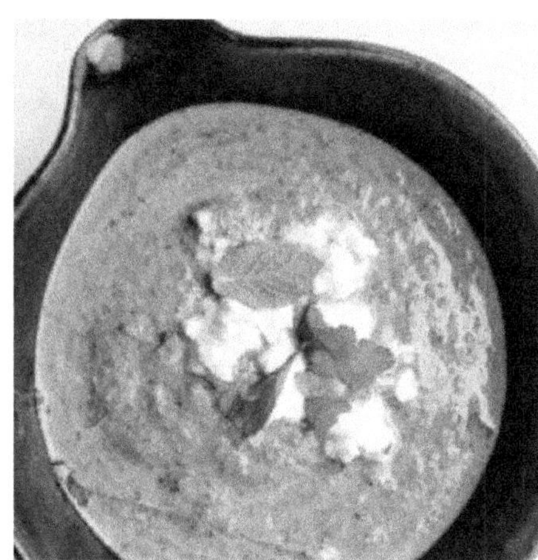

SPINACH PUREE AND SWISS CHARD

Serves: 8
Prep time: 25 minutes

Ingredients

- ½ pound swiss chard
- 1-pound baby spinach leaves
- 1 cup cauliflower florets
- 1 leek
- 4 tablespoons extra virgin olive oil
- 3 cups water
- ¼ cup cream cheese
- Salt and pepper to taste

Directions

1. Rinse the leek. Cut into thick slices.
2. Heat olive oil. Add the cauliflower and leek. Cook for 3 minutes.
3. Add spinach leaves, swiss chard, salt and pepper. Simmer 15 minutes.
4. Allow the vegetables to cool down, 10 minutes. Transfer to food processor. Blend until smooth.
5. Return the soup to the pan and put back on the heat. Stir in the cream cheese and water. Heat 5 minutes.
6. Pour into bowls. Serve.

Nutritional Value (Amount per Serving)

Protein: 3 g
Carbs: 8.7 g
Fat: 2.8 g

DINNER RECIPE

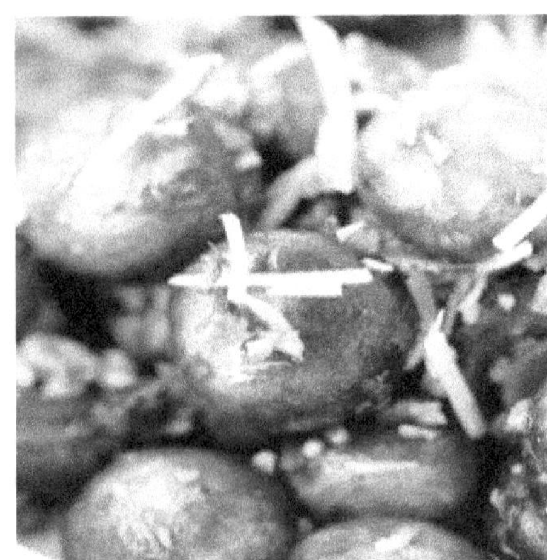

Mushrooms Roasted with Herbs & Parmesan

Serves: 6
Prep time: 35 minutes

Ingredients

- 1 pound Cremini mushrooms
- 1 can diced tomatoes
- 2 cups grated Parmesan cheese
- 2 tablespoons ghee
- 2 tablespoons mashed garlic
- 1 tablespoon fresh parsley
- 2 tablespoons fresh basil
- 1 tablespoon fresh thyme
- Salt and pepper to taste

Directions

1. The oven to be preheated to 400°F. Rinse the mushrooms, pat dry. Slice off stems.
2. In a large non-stick, oven-safe frying pan, melt the ghee.
3. Sauté the mushrooms for 5 minutes. Season with salt and pepper.
4. In a medium bowl, combine the herbs, tomatoes, salt and pepper. Stir mixture in with mushrooms. Sprinkle Parmesan cheese over top. Bake 25 minutes.
5. Remove from oven. Divide on plates. Serve.

Nutritional Value (Amount per Serving)

Protein: 14.8 g
Carbs: 5.3 g
Fat: 9.7 g

Day 16

Shopping list

- Tofu
- Non-dairy milk
- Onion
- Jalapeno
- Tomatoes
- Cilantro
- Potato
- Tortilla wraps
- Chili powder
- Salt and pepper
- Lemon juice
- Lime juice
- Clove garlic
- Avocado
- Black beans
- Cumin
- Chili powder
- Garlic powder
- Portobello mushroom caps
- Red bell pepper
- Orange bell pepper
- Salt and pepper
- Virgin olive oil
- Spinach
- Potatoes
- Spinach
- Parsley
- Carrots
- Vegetable broth

BREAKFAST RECIPE

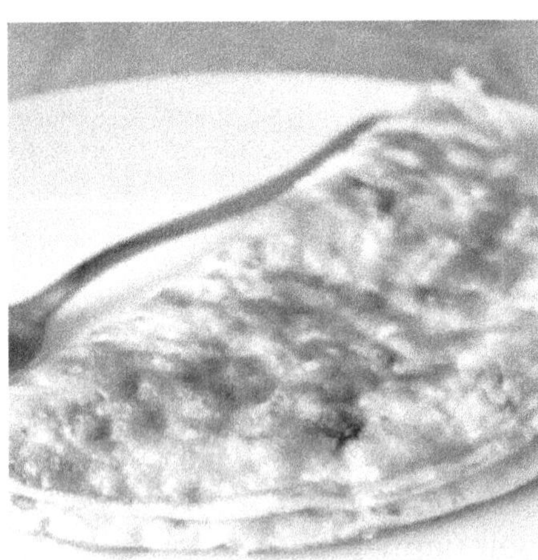

FETA MINTY OMELETTE

Serves: 2
Prep time: 15 minutes

Ingredients

- 3 large eggs
- 6 mint leaves
- 4 ounces' feta cheese
- Salt and pepper to taste
- Olive oil for frying

Directions

1. The oven to be preheated to 400 ℉.

2. In a medium bowl, combine eggs, feta cheese, mint leaves, salt and pepper. Whisk thoroughly.

3. In a non-stick, oven-safe frying pan, heat up some olive oil (a light layer drizzled over the bottom). Pour the egg mixture into the frying pan. Cook for 3 minutes.

4. Remove frying pan from stove and place in the oven. Cook 5 minutes.

5. Transfer omelette to a plate. Serve.

Nutrition Value (Amount per Serving)

Protein: 9.9 g
Carbs: 0.8 g
Fat: 7.6 g

LUNCH RECIPE

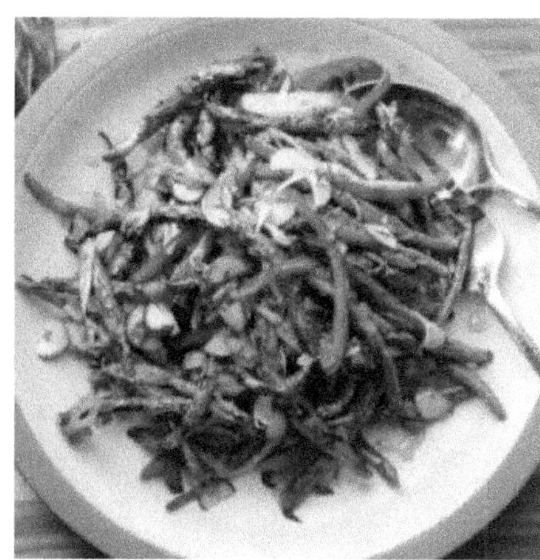

Pressure-Cooker Greens and Red-Hot Salad

Serves: 6
Prep time: 15 minutes

Ingredients

- 1½ pounds red cabbage, sliced into small wedges
- 1½ pounds Brussels sprouts, sliced into small wedges
- 3 medium beets, sliced into small wedges
- 8 cloves garlic, minced
- 3 tablespoons olive oil
- 1 tablespoon finely chopped fresh thyme

Directions

1. Place the vegetables and garlic in a pressure cooker.
2. Add the salt, pepper, thyme, and oil. Stir.
3. Set the cooker on Sauté. Cook for 15 minutes on high pressure.
4. Once ready, select natural release. Allow the pressure to go down naturally. (Approximately 15 - 20 minutes.)
5. Transfer vegetables to a platter. Serve.

Nutritional Value (Amount per Serving)

Protein: 6.5 g
Carbs: 13.4 g
Fat: 7.3 g

DINNER RECIPE

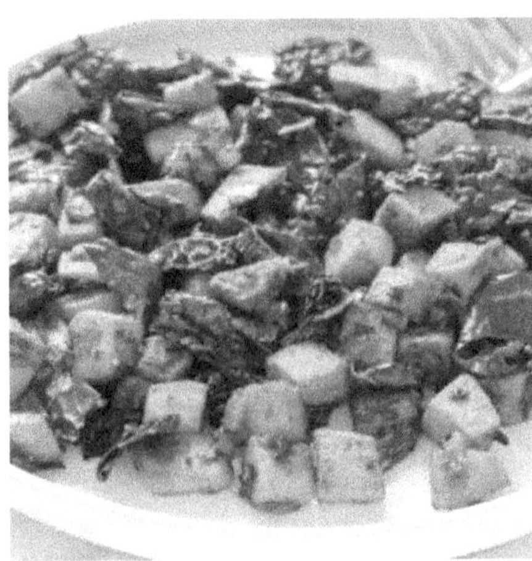

EGG WITH POWER GREENS AND SWEET POTATO CASSEROLE

Serves: 4
Prep time: 1 hour and 10 minutes

Ingredients

- 8 large eggs
- ½ teaspoon coconut oil
- 4 cups power greens (spinach, kale, arugula)
- 2 peeled sweet potatoes, diced
- 1 green onion, chopped
- ¼ cup coconut milk
- 1 teaspoon garlic powder
- ¼ teaspoon nutmeg
- Salt and pepper to taste
- Seasoning blend of your choice

Directions

1. Preheat oven to 400° F. Grease a casserole dish with coconut oil.
2. In a large bowl, whisk the eggs. Add the green onion, sweet potato, coconut milk, power greens and seasoning. Pour the egg mixture into the casserole.
3. Place dish in the oven. Bake 45 minutes.
4. Remove dish from the oven. Cover with foil. Bake for 15 more minutes.
5. Remove from oven. Cut into pieces and serve.

Nutritional Value (Amount per Serving)

Protein: 13.8 g
Carbs: 10.8 g
Fat: 11.9 g

Day 17

Shopping list

- Tofu
- Non-dairy milk
- Onion
- Jalapeno
- Tomatoes
- Cilantro
- Potato
- Tortilla wraps
- Chili powder
- Salt and pepper
- Lemon juice
- Lime juice
- Clove garlic
- Avocado
- Black beans
- Cumin
- Chili powder
- Garlic powder
- Portobello mushroom caps
- Red bell pepper
- Orange bell pepper
- Salt and pepper
- Virgin olive oil
- Spinach
- Potatoes
- Spinach
- Parsley
- Carrots
- Vegetable broth

BREAKFAST RECIPE

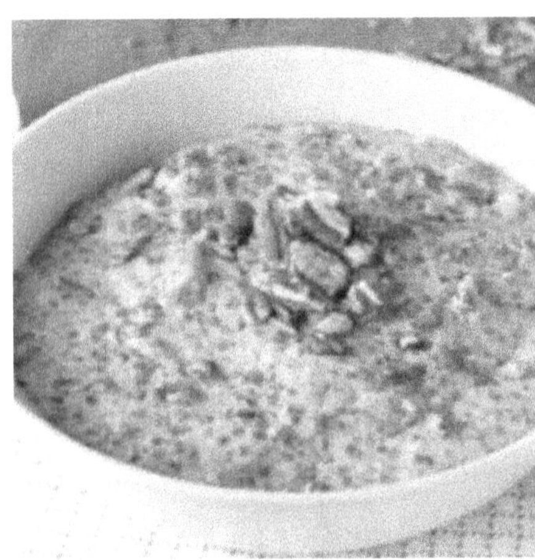

FLAX MEAL CINNAMON PORRIDGE

Serves: 1
Prep time: 5 minutes

Ingredients

- 4 tablespoons soft cream cheese
- 4 tablespoons flax meal
- 1 cup water
- 1 cup sweetener
- Ground cinnamon to taste

Directions

1. Add all of the ingredients. Stir well.
2. Microwave for 2 minutes. Stir again. Top with fresh berries.
3. Serve.

Nutritional Value (Amount per Serving)

Protein: 3.4 g
Carbs: 6 g
Fat: 10.5 g

LUNCH RECIPE

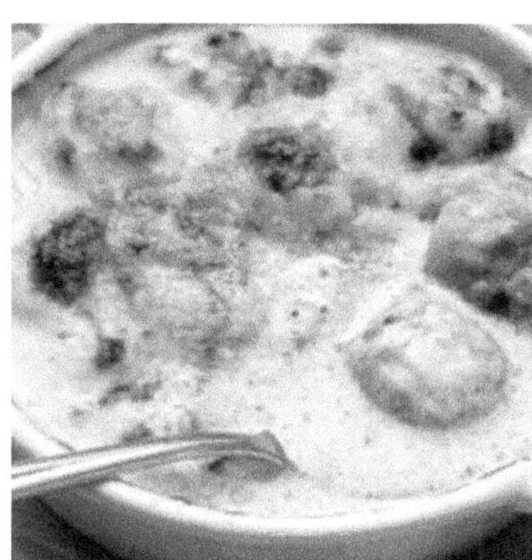

CREAMY CHEESY BRUSSELS SPROUTS

Serves: 2
Prep time: 15 minutes

Ingredients

- 25 Brussels sprouts
- 4 cloves garlic, minced
- ¾ cup cream cheese
- 2 tablespoons extra virgin olive oil
- 2 teaspoons organic fresh lemon juice
- Salt and pepper to taste

Directions

1. Rinse the Brussels sprouts in cold water. Remove the stems.
2. Heat olive oil.
3. Add the minced garlic and Brussels sprouts to the pan. Sauté until tender.
4. Stir in the cream cheese and lemon juice.
5. Transfer to bowls. Serve.

Nutritional Value (Amount per Serving)

Protein: 11.7 g
Carbs: 18.5 g
Fat: 9.8 g

DINNER RECIPE

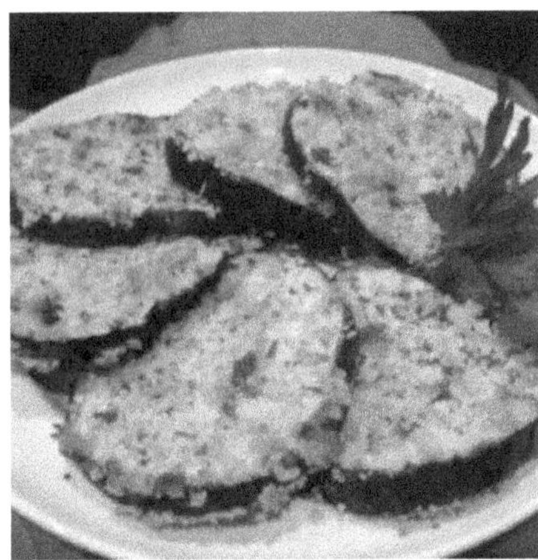

CHEESY FRIED EGGPLANT SLICES

Serves: 6
Prep time: 20 minutes

Ingredients

- 1 eggplant
- 1 large egg
- 1 cup almond flour
- 1 cup grated Parmesan cheese
- ½ cup coconut oil or butter
- Garlic powder
- Salt and pepper to taste

Directions

1. Rinse the eggplant and pat dry. Cut into slices, ½ inch thick. Arrange on a plate.

2. Sprinkle with salt. Let sit for 30 minutes.

3. Whisk the egg. Combine Parmesan cheese, garlic powder, almond flour, salt and pepper. Stir well.

4. Heat butter.

5. Fry until crispy and golden brown.

6. Place the cooked eggplant on a paper towel-lined plate to drain excess oil. Repeat with remaining eggplant slices.

7. Serve.

Nutritional Value (Amount per Serving)

Protein: 13.2 g
Carbs: 7.9 g
Fat: 33 g

Day 18

Shopping list

- Tofu
- Non-dairy milk
- Onion
- Jalapeno
- Tomatoes
- Cilantro
- Potato
- Tortilla wraps
- Chili powder
- Salt and pepper
- Lemon juice
- Lime juice
- Clove garlic
- Avocado
- Black beans
- Cumin
- Chili powder
- Garlic powder
- Portobello mushroom caps
- Red bell pepper
- Orange bell pepper
- Salt and pepper
- Virgin olive oil
- Spinach
- Potatoes
- Spinach
- Parsley
- Carrots
- Vegetable broth

BREAKFAST RECIPE

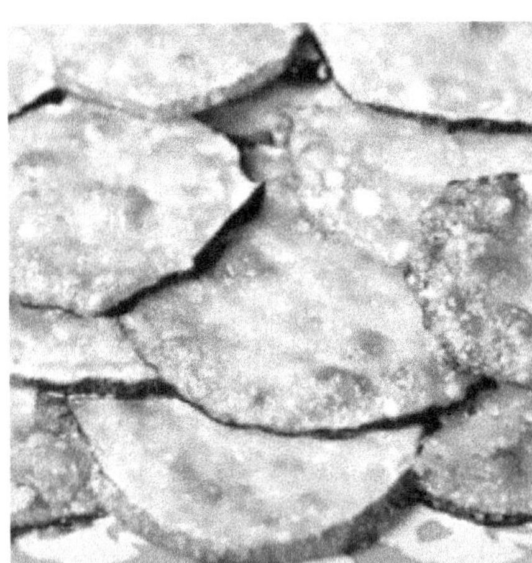

BAKED ZUCCHINI PARMIGIANINO

Serves: 6
Prep Time: 40 minutes

Ingredients

- 3 large eggs
- 1 cup almond flour
- 1 cup ground almonds
- 2 zucchinis, thinly sliced
- 1 cup Parmigiano-Reggiano cheese, grated
- 1 teaspoon dried oregano
- Salt and pepper to taste

Directions

1. The oven to be preheated to 400　F.

2. In a large bowl combine the oregano and Parmigiano-Reggiano cheese. Season with salt and pepper to taste. Set aside.

3. Pour the almond flour into a separate bowl.

4. In a third bowl, whisk the eggs together. Season with salt and pepper to taste.

5. Dip sliced zucchini in flour, then in the egg mixture, then in the almond flour.

6. Bake 30 minutes. Serve.

Nutritional Value (Amount per Serving)

Protein: 14.1 g
Carbs: 13.8 g
Fat: 17.5 g

LUNCH RECIPE

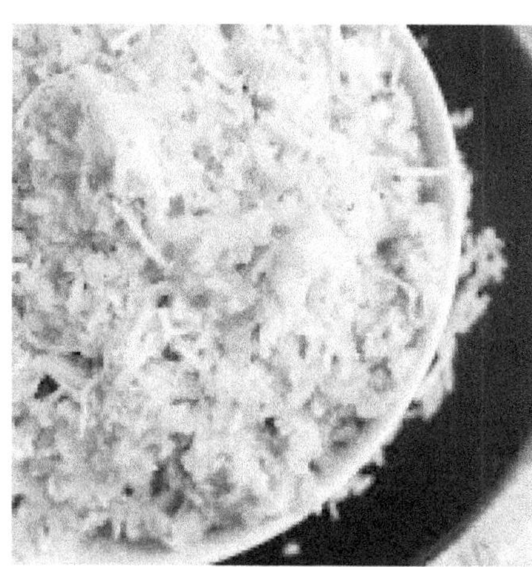

Cauliflower Coconut Rice

Serves: 3
Prep Time: 20 minutes

Ingredients

- 3 cups cauliflower rice
- ½ tsp onion powder
- 1 tsp chili paste
- 2/3 cup coconut milk
- Salt

Directions

1. Add all ingredients to the pan and heat over medium-low heat. Stir to combine.
2. Cook for 10 minutes. Stir after every 2 minutes.
3. Remove lid and cook until excess liquid absorbed.
4. Serve and enjoy.

Nutritional Value (Amount per Serving)

Protein: 3.4 g
Carbs: 9.2 g
Fat: 13.1 g
Sugar: 4.8 g
Calories: 155
Cholesterol: 1 mg

DINNER RECIPE

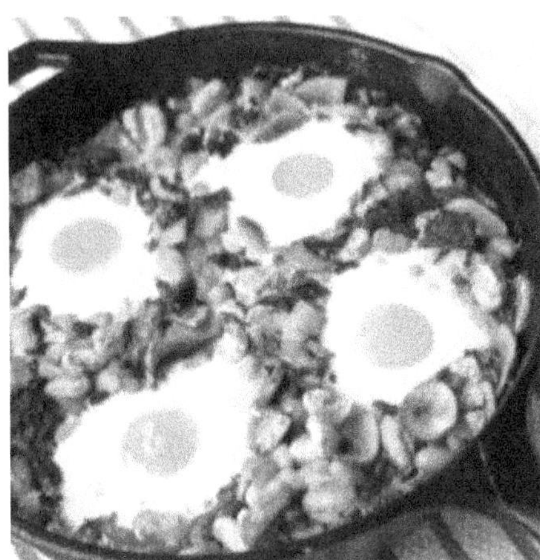

BROILED EGGS

Serves: 2
Prep Time: 20 minutes

Ingredients

- 4 large eggs
- 6 tablespoons heavy cream
- 1 tablespoon extra-virgin olive oil
- 1 tablespoon Parmesan cheese, plus extra for serving
- ¼ cup button mushrooms, sliced
- ¼ cup baby spinach
- 1 pinch red pepper flakes
- Salt and pepper to taste

Directions

1. Preheat broiler to 400   F. Rinse mushrooms, pat dry.
2. In a large non-stick, oven-safe frying pan, heat the oil over medium heat. Fry the eggs on one side for 3 minutes. Remove to a plate and set aside.
3. Pour half the heavy cream in the pan. Add the mushrooms. Simmer for 3 minutes.
4. Stir in the remaining heavy cream. Add the Parmesan cheese. Stir well.
5. Place under broiler for 3 minutes.
6. Pull the pan out of the oven. Add the spinach leaves and red pepper flakes. Stir well.
7. Return the eggs to the pan. Return the pan to the broiler for 2-3 minutes.
8. Remove the pan from the oven. Sprinkle more Parmesan cheese over top.
9. Garnish with fresh spinach leaves. Serve.

Nutritional Value (Amount per Serving)

Protein: 8.5 g
Carbs: 2.8 g
Fat: 20.9 g

Day 19

Shopping list

- Tofu
- Non-dairy milk
- Onion
- Jalapeno
- Tomatoes
- Cilantro
- Potato
- Tortilla wraps
- Chili powder
- Salt and pepper
- Lemon juice
- Lime juice
- Clove garlic
- Avocado
- Black beans
- Cumin
- Chili powder
- Garlic powder
- Portobello mushroom caps
- Red bell pepper
- Orange bell pepper
- Salt and pepper
- Virgin olive oil
- Spinach
- Potatoes
- Spinach
- Parsley
- Carrots
- Vegetable broth

BREAKFAST RECIPE

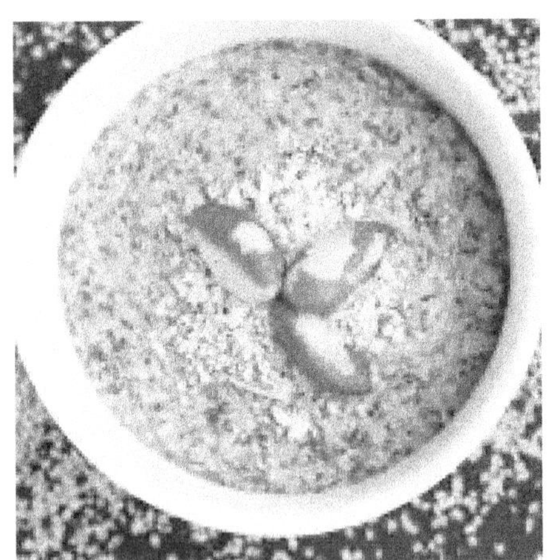

ALMOND HEMP HEART PORRIDGE

Serves: 2
Prep Time: 10 minutes

Ingredients:

- ¼ cup almond flour
- ½ tsp cinnamon
- ¾ tsp vanilla extract
- 5 drops stevia
- 1 tbsp chia seeds
- 2 tbsp ground flax seed
- ½ cup hemp hearts
- 1 cup unsweetened coconut milk

Directions:

1. Add all ingredients except almond flour to a saucepan. Stir to combine.
2. Heat over medium heat until just starts to lightly boil.
3. Once start bubbling then stir well and cook for 1 minute more.
4. Remove from heat and stir in almond flour.

Nutritional Value (Amount per Serving)

Protein: 16.2 g
Carbs: 9.2 g
Fat: 24.4 g
Sugar: 1.8 g
Calories: 329
Cholesterol: 0 mg

LUNCH RECIPE

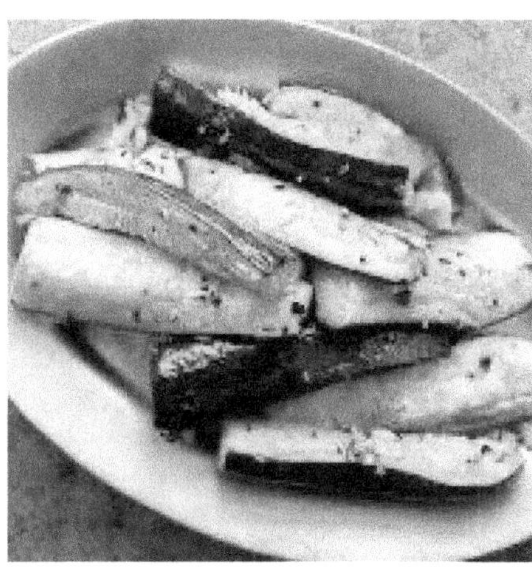

GARLIC ZUCCHINI SQUASH

Serves: 4
Prep Time: 20 minutes

Ingredients

- 1 small squash, sliced
- 2 tbsp fresh basil, chopped
- 2 tbsp olive oil
- 1 garlic clove, chopped
- 1 large onion, sliced
- 2 fresh tomatoes, cut into wedges
- 1 small zucchini, sliced
- Pepper
- Salt

Directions

1. Heat olive oil.
2. Add onion, squash, zucchini, and garlic and sauté until lightly brown.
3. Add basil and tomatoes and cook for 5 minutes. Season with pepper and salt.
4. Simmer over low heat until squash is tender.
5. Stir well and serve.

Nutritional Value (Amount per Serving)

Protein: 1.4 g
Carbs: 8.2 g
Fat: 7.2 g
Sugar: 4.4 g
Calories: 97;
Cholesterol: 0 mg;

DINNER RECIPE

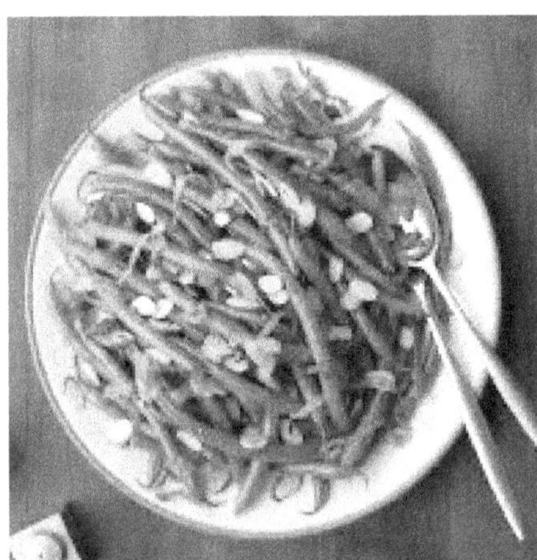

ALMOND GREEN BEANS

Serves: 4
Prep Time: 20 minutes

Ingredients:

- 1 lb fresh green beans, trimmed
- 1/3 cup almonds, sliced
- 4 garlic cloves, sliced
- 2 tbsp olive oil
- 1 tbsp lemon juice
- ½ tsp sea salt

Directions:

1. Add green beans, salt, and lemon juice in a mixing bowl. Toss well and set aside.
2. Heat oil in a pan over medium heat.
3. Add sliced almonds and sauté until lightly browned.
4. Add garlic and sauté for 30 seconds.
5. Pour almond mixture over green beans and toss well.
6. Stir well and serve immediately.

Nutritional Value (Amount per Serving)

Protein: 4 g
Carbs: 10.9 g
Fat: 11.2 g
Sugar: 2 g
Calories: 146
Cholesterol: 0 mg;

Day 20

Shopping list

- Tofu
- Non-dairy milk
- Onion
- Jalapeno
- Tomatoes
- Cilantro
- Potato
- Tortilla wraps
- Chili powder
- Salt and pepper
- Lemon juice
- Lime juice
- Clove garlic
- Avocado
- Black beans
- Cumin
- Chili powder
- Garlic powder
- Portobello mushroom caps
- Red bell pepper
- Orange bell pepper
- Salt and pepper
- Virgin olive oil
- Spinach
- Potatoes
- Spinach
- Parsley
- Carrots
- Vegetable broth

BREAKFAST RECIPE

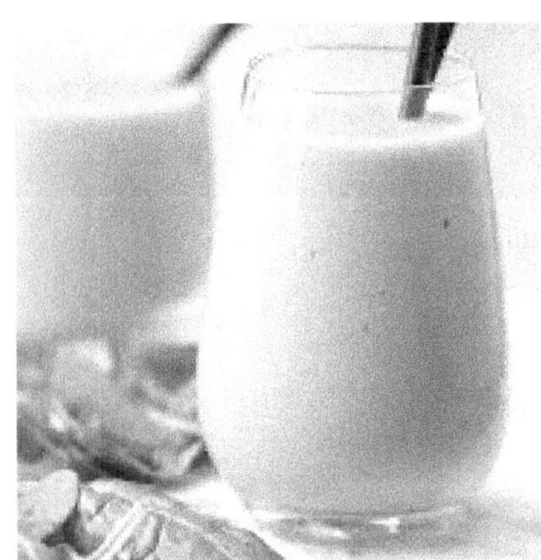

Healthy Spinach Green Smoothie

Serves: 1
Prep Time: 5 minutes

Ingredients

- 1 cup ice cube
- 2/3 cup water
- ½ cup unsweetened almond milk
- 5 drops liquid stevia
- ½ tsp matcha powder
- 1 tsp vanilla extract
- 1 tbsp MCT oil
- ½ avocado
- 2/3 cup spinach

Directions

1. Blend until smooth and creamy then serve.

Nutritional Value (Amount per Serving)

Protein: 1.6 g
Carbs: 3.8 g
Fat: 18.3 g
Sugar: 0.6 g
Calories: 167
Cholesterol: 0 mg

LUNCH RECIPE

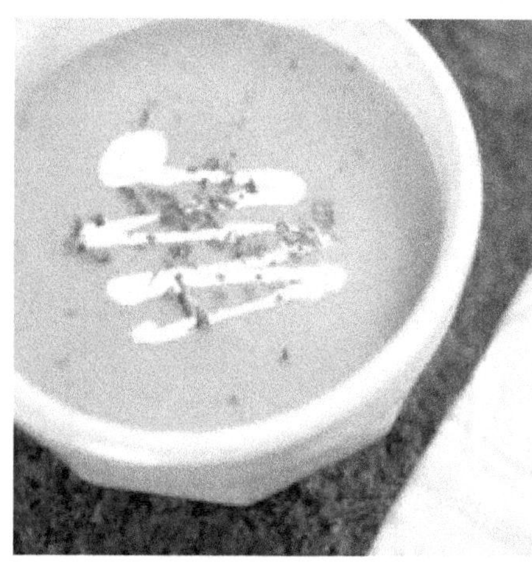

Creamy Squash Soup

Serves: 8
Prep Time: 35 minutes

Ingredients

- 3 cups butternut squash, chopped
- 1 ½ cups unsweetened coconut milk
- 1 tbsp coconut oil
- 1 tsp dried onion flakes
- 1 tbsp curry powder
- 4 cups water
- 1 garlic clove
- 1 tsp kosher salt

Directions

1. Add squash, coconut oil, onion flakes, curry powder, water, garlic, and salt into a large saucepan. Bring to boil over high heat.
2. Simmer for 20 minutes.
3. Puree the soup using a blender until smooth. Cook for 2 minutes.
4. Stir well and serve hot.

Nutritional Value (Amount per Serving)

Protein: 1.7 g
Carbs: 9.4 g
Fat: 12.6 g
Sugar: 2.8 g
Calories: 146
Cholesterol: 0 mg

DINNER RECIPE

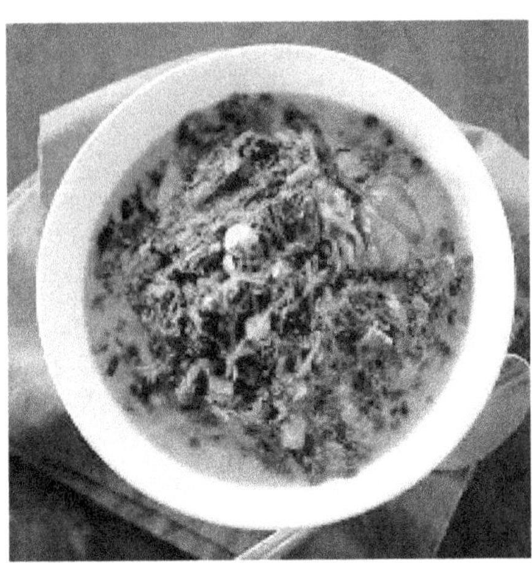

SPINACH WITH COCONUT MILK

Serves: 6
Prep Time: 25 minutes

Ingredients

- 16 oz spinach
- 2 tsp curry powder
- 13.5 oz coconut milk
- 1 tsp lemon zest
- ½ tsp salt

Directions

1. Add spinach in pan and heat over medium heat. Once it is hot then add curry paste and few tablespoons of coconut milk. Stir well.

2. Add remaining coconut milk, lemon zest, and salt and cook until thickened.

3. Serve and enjoy.

Nutritional Value (Amount per Serving)

Protein: 3.7 g
Carbs: 6.7 g
Fat: 15.6 g
Sugar: 2.5 g
Calories: 167
Cholesterol: 0 mg

Day 21

Shopping list

- Tofu
- Non-dairy milk
- Onion
- Jalapeno
- Tomatoes
- Cilantro
- Potato
- Tortilla wraps
- Chili powder
- Salt and pepper
- Lemon juice
- Lime juice
- Clove garlic
- Avocado
- Black beans
- Cumin
- Chili powder
- Garlic powder
- Portobello mushroom caps
- Red bell pepper
- Orange bell pepper
- Salt and pepper
- Virgin olive oil
- Spinach
- Potatoes
- Spinach
- Parsley
- Carrots
- Vegetable broth

BREAKFAST RECIPE

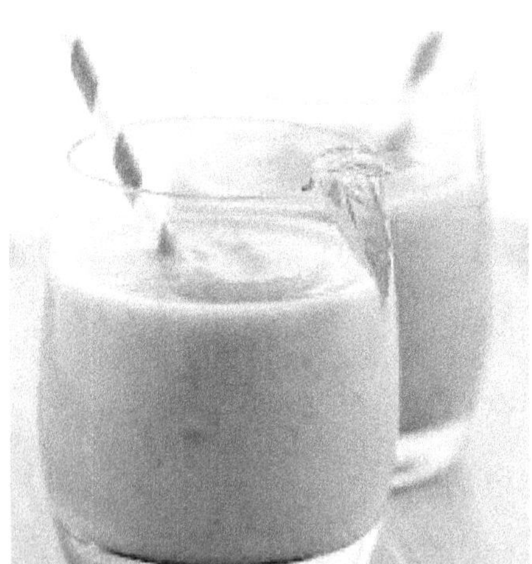

Apple Avocado Coconut Smoothie

Serves: 2
Prep Time: 5 minutes

Ingredients

- 1 tsp coconut oil
- 1 tbsp collagen powder
- 1 tbsp fresh lime juice

- ½ cup unsweetened coconut milk
- ¼ apple, slice
- 1 avocado

Directions

1. Blend until smooth and creamy.
2. Serve and enjoy.

Nutritional Value (Amount per Serving)

Protein: 2 g
Carbs: 13.6 g
Fat: 23.9 g
Sugar: 3.4 g
Cholesterol: 0 mg

LUNCH RECIPE

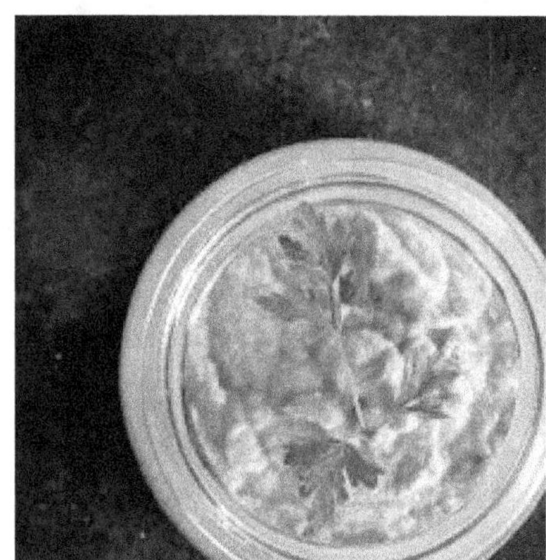

Asparagus Mash

Serves: 2
Prep Time: 20 minutes

Ingredients

- 10 asparagus shoots, chopped
- 1 tsp lemon juice
- 2 tbsp fresh parsley
- 2 tbsp coconut cream
- 1 small onion, diced
- 1 tbsp coconut oil
- Pepper
- Salt

Directions

1. Sauté onion in coconut oil until onion is softened.
2. Blanch chopped asparagus in hot water for 2 minutes and drain immediately.
3. Add sautéed onion, lemon juice, parsley, coconut cream, asparagus, pepper, and salt and blend until smooth.
4. Serve warm and enjoy.

Nutritional Value (Amount per Serving)

Protein: 2.6 g
Carbs: 7.5 g
Fat: 10.6 g
Sugar: 3.6 g
Calories: 125
Cholesterol: 0 mg

DINNER RECIPE

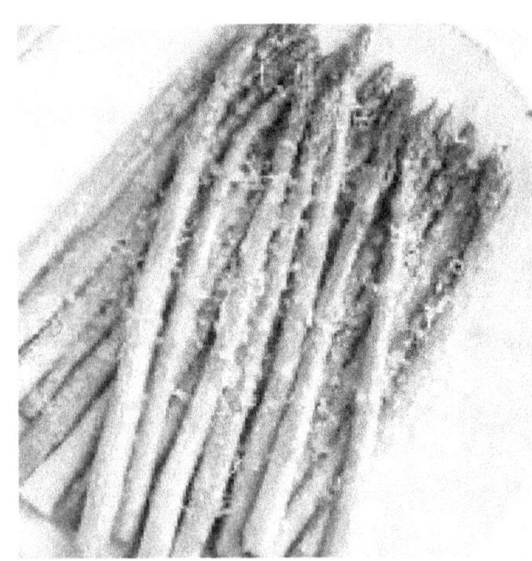

BAKED ASPARAGUS

Serves: 4
Prep Time: 25 minutes

Ingredients

- 40 asparagus spears
- 2 tbsp vegetable seasoning
- 2 tbsp garlic powder
- 2 tbsp salt

Directions

1. The oven to be preheated to 450 F/ 232 C.

2. Arrange all asparagus spears on baking tray and season with vegetable seasoning, garlic powder, and salt.

3. Bake for 20 minutes.

4. Serve warm and enjoy.

Nutritional Value (Amount per Serving)

Protein: 6.7 g
Carbs: 13.5 g
Fat: 0.9 g
Sugar: 5.5 g
Calories: 75
Cholesterol: 0 mg

Day 22

Shopping list

- Tofu
- Non-dairy milk
- Onion
- Jalapeno
- Tomatoes
- Cilantro
- Potato
- Tortilla wraps
- Chili powder
- Salt and pepper
- Lemon juice
- Lime juice
- Clove garlic
- Avocado
- Black beans
- Cumin
- Chili powder
- Garlic powder
- Portobello mushroom caps
- Red bell pepper
- Orange bell pepper
- Salt and pepper
- Virgin olive oil
- Spinach
- Potatoes
- Spinach
- Parsley
- Carrots
- Vegetable broth

BREAKFAST RECIPE

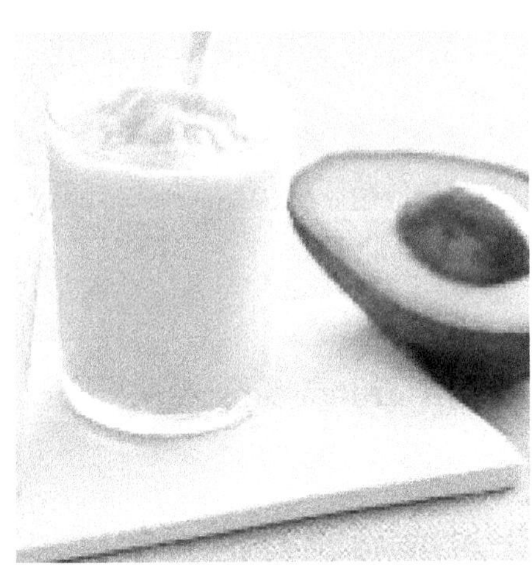

Avocado Breakfast Smoothie

Serves: 2
Prep Time: 5 minutes

Ingredients

- 5 drops liquid stevia
- ¼ cup ice cubes
- ½ avocado
- 1 tsp vanilla extract
- 1 cup unsweetened coconut milk

Directions

1. Blend until smooth and creamy.
2. Serve immediately and enjoy.

Nutritional Value (Amount per Serving)

Protein: 1 g
Carbs: 5.6 g
Fat: 11.8 g
Sugar: 0.5 g
Calories: 131
Cholesterol: 0 mg

LUNCH RECIPE

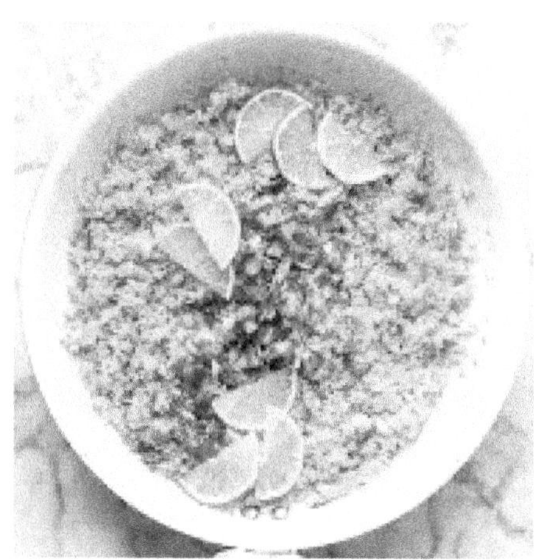

Mexican Cauliflower Rice

Serves: 4
Prep Time: 25 minutes

Ingredients

- 1 medium cauliflower head, cut into florets
- ½ cup tomato sauce
- ¼ tsp black pepper
- 1 tsp chili powder
- 2 garlic cloves, minced
- ½ medium onion, diced
- 1 tbsp coconut oil
- ½ tsp sea salt

Directions

1. Add cauliflower florets into the food processor and process until it looks like rice.
2. Heat oil in a pan over medium-high heat.
3. Add onion to the pan and sauté for 5 minutes or until softened.
4. Add garlic and cook for 1 minute.
5. Add cauliflower rice, chili powder, pepper, and salt. Stir well.
6. Cook for 5 minutes.
7. Stir well and serve warm.

Nutritional Value (Amount per Serving)

Protein: 3.6 g
Carbs: 11.5 g
Fat: 3.7g
Sugar: 5.4 g
Calories: 83
Cholesterol: 0 mg;

DINNER RECIPE

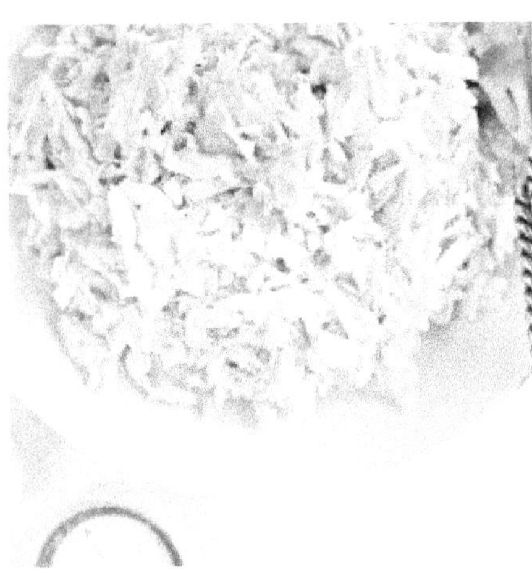

Classic Cabbage Slaw

Serves: 3
Prep Time: 20 minutes

Ingredients

- 4 cups green cabbage, shredded
- 2 garlic cloves
- 1 tbsp sesame oil
- 2 tbsp tamari
- 1 tsp vinegar
- 1 tsp chili paste
- ½ cup macadamia nuts, chopped

Directions

1. Toss shredded green cabbage in a pan with chili paste, sesame oil, vinegar, and tamari on medium-low heat.

2. Add garlic and cook for 5 minutes or until cabbage is softened.

3. Stir everything well. Add macadamia nuts and cook for 5 minutes.

4. Stir well and serve.

Nutritional Value (Amount per Serving)

Protein: 4.5 g
Carbs: 10.5 g
Fat: 21.8 g
Sugar: 4.7 g
Calories: 240
Cholesterol: 1 mg

Day 23

Shopping list

- Tofu
- Non-dairy milk
- Onion
- Jalapeno
- Tomatoes
- Cilantro
- Potato
- Tortilla wraps
- Chili powder
- Salt and pepper
- Lemon juice
- Lime juice
- Clove garlic
- Avocado
- Black beans
- Cumin
- Chili powder
- Garlic powder
- Portobello mushroom caps
- Red bell pepper
- Orange bell pepper
- Salt and pepper
- Virgin olive oil
- Spinach
- Potatoes
- Spinach
- Parsley
- Carrots
- Vegetable broth

BREAKFAST RECIPE

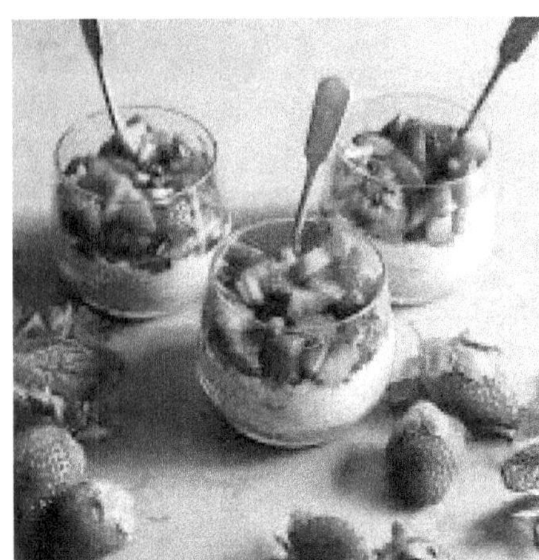

Strawberry Chia Matcha Pudding

Serves: 1
Prep Time: 10 minutes

Ingredients

- 5 drops liquid stevia
- 2 strawberries, diced
- 1 ½ tbsp chia seeds
- ¾ cup unsweetened coconut milk
- ½ tsp matcha powder

Directions

1. Add all ingredients except strawberries into the glass jar and mix well.
2. Close jar with lid and place in refrigerator for 4 hours.
3. Add strawberries into the pudding and mix well.
4. Serve and enjoy.

Nutritional Value (Amount per Serving)

Protein: 2.5 g
Carbs: 5.6 g
Fat: 6.5 g
Sugar: 1.2 g
Calories: 93
Cholesterol: 0 mg

LUNCH RECIPE

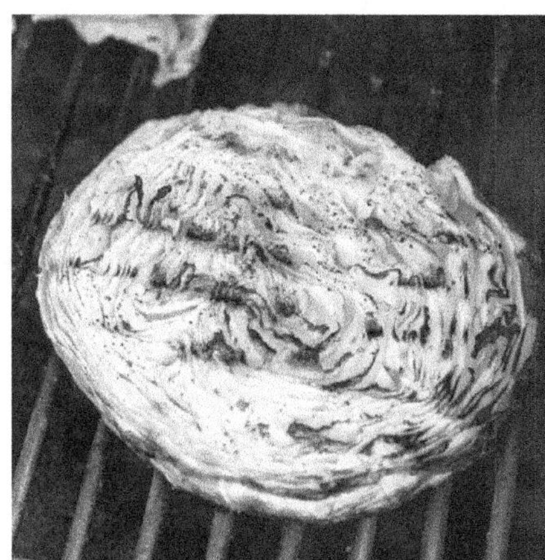

Delicious Cabbage Steaks

Serves: 6
Prep Time: 1 hour and 20 minutes

Ingredients

- 1 medium cabbage head, slice 1" thick
- 2 tbsp olive oil
- 1 tbsp garlic, minced
- Pepper
- Salt

Directions

1. Mix together garlic and olive oil.

2. Brush garlic and olive oil mixture onto both sides of sliced cabbage.

3. Season cabbage slices with pepper and salt.

4. Place cabbage slices onto a baking tray and bake at 350 F/ 180 C for 1 hour. Turn after 30 minutes.

5. Serve and enjoy.

Nutritional Value (Amount per Serving)

Protein: 1.6 g
Carbs: 7.4 g
Fat: 4.8 g
Sugar: 3.8 g
Calories: 72
Cholesterol: 0 mg

DINNER RECIPE

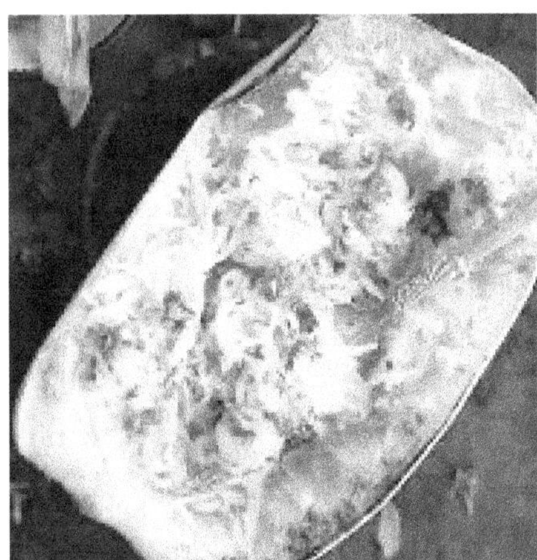

HERB SPAGHETTI SQUASH

Serves: 4
Prep Time: 30 minutes

Ingredients

- 4 cups spaghetti squash, cooked
- ½ tsp pepper
- ½ tsp sage
- 1 tsp dried parsley
- 1 tsp dried thyme
- 1 tsp dried rosemary
- 1 tsp garlic powder
- 2 tbsp olive oil
- 1 tsp salt

Directions

1. The oven to be preheated to 350 F/ 180 C.
2. Mix well to combine.
3. Transfer bowl mixture to the oven safe dish and cook in preheated oven for 15 minutes.
4. Stir well and serve.

Nutritional Value (Amount per Serving)

Protein: 0.9 g
Carbs: 8.1 g
Fat: 7.7 g
Sugar: 0.2 g
Calories: 96
Cholesterol: 0 mg

Day 24

Shopping list

- Tofu
- Non-dairy milk
- Onion
- Jalapeno
- Tomatoes
- Cilantro
- Potato
- Tortilla wraps
- Chili powder
- Salt and pepper
- Lemon juice
- Lime juice
- Clove garlic
- Avocado
- Black beans
- Cumin
- Chili powder
- Garlic powder
- Portobello mushroom caps
- Red bell pepper
- Orange bell pepper
- Salt and pepper
- Virgin olive oil
- Spinach
- Potatoes
- Spinach
- Parsley
- Carrots
- Vegetable broth

BREAKFAST RECIPE

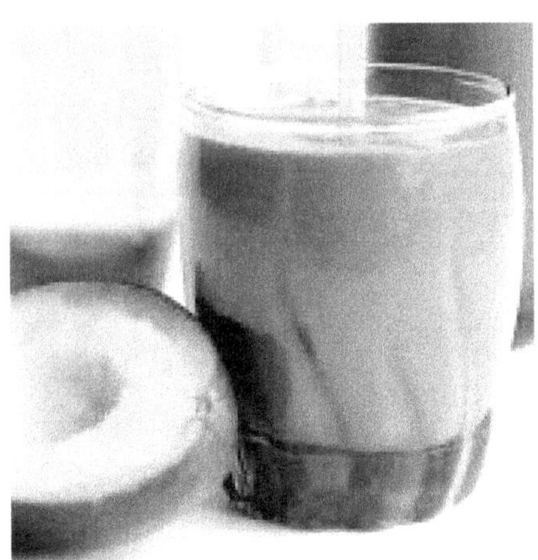

Avocado Chocó Cinnamon Smoothie

Serves: 1
Prep Time: 5 minutes

Ingredients

- ½ tsp coconut oil
- 5 drops liquid stevia
- ¼ tsp vanilla extract
- 1 tsp ground cinnamon
- 2 tsp unsweetened cocoa powder
- ½ avocado
- ¾ cup unsweetened coconut milk

Directions

1. Add all ingredients blend until smooth and creamy.
2. Serve immediately and enjoy.

Nutritional Value (Amount per Serving)

Protein: 1.2 g
Carbs: 5.1 g
Fat: 8.3 g
Sugar: 0.2 g
Calories: 95
Cholesterol: 0 mg

LUNCH RECIPE

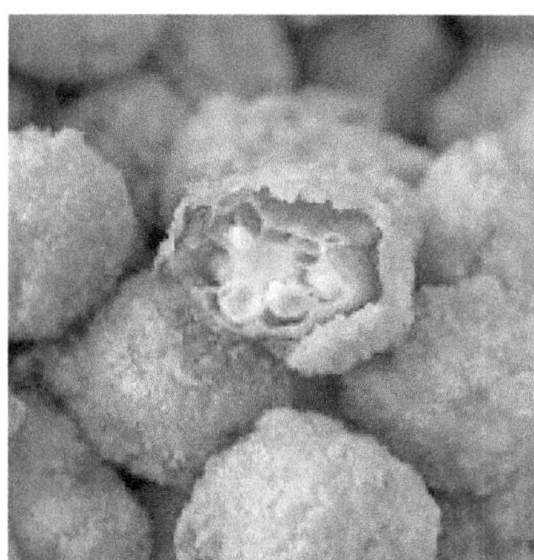

FRIED OKRA

Serves: 4
Prep Time: 20 minutes

Ingredients

- 1 lb fresh okra, cut into ¼" slices
- 1/3 cup almond meal
- Pepper
- Salt
- Oil for frying

Directions

1. Heat oil.
2. In a bowl, mix together sliced okra, almond meal, pepper, and salt until well coated.
3. Once the oil is hot then add okra to the hot oil and cook until lightly browned.
4. Remove fried okra from pan and allow to drain on paper towels.
5. Serve and enjoy.

Nutritional Value (Amount per Serving)

Protein: 3.9 g
Carbs: 10.2 g
Fat: 4.2 g
Sugar: 10.2 g
Calories: 91
Cholesterol: 0 mg

DINNER RECIPE

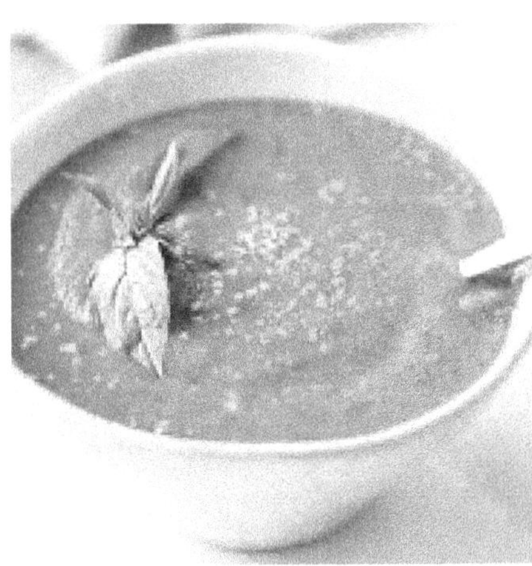

Basil Tomato Soup

Serves: 6
Prep Time: 20 minutes

Ingredients

- 28 oz can tomatoes
- ¼ cup basil pesto
- ¼ tsp dried basil leaves
- 1 tsp apple cider vinegar
- 2 tbsp erythritol
- ¼ tsp garlic powder
- ½ tsp onion powder
- 2 cups water
- 1 ½ tsp kosher salt

Directions

1. Add tomatoes, garlic powder, onion powder, water, and salt in a saucepan.
2. Bring to boil over medium heat. Reduce heat and simmer for 2 minutes.
3. Heat and blend until smooth.
4. Stir in pesto, dried basil, vinegar, and erythritol.
5. Stir well and serve warm.

Nutritional Value (Amount per Serving)

Protein: 1.3 g
Carbs: 12.2 g
Fat: 0 g
Sugar: 9.6 g
Calories: 30
Cholesterol: 0 mg

Day 25

Shopping list

- Tofu
- Non-dairy milk
- Onion
- Jalapeno
- Tomatoes
- Cilantro
- Potato
- Tortilla wraps
- Chili powder
- Salt and pepper
- Lemon juice
- Lime juice
- Clove garlic
- Avocado
- Black beans
- Cumin
- Chili powder
- Garlic powder
- Portobello mushroom caps
- Red bell pepper
- Orange bell pepper
- Salt and pepper
- Virgin olive oil
- Spinach
- Potatoes
- Spinach
- Parsley
- Carrots
- Vegetable broth

BREAKFAST RECIPE

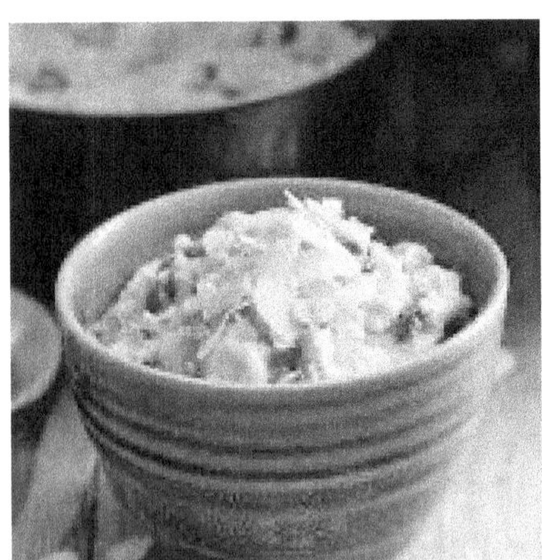

ALMOND COCONUT PORRIDGE

Serves: 2
Prep Time: 10 minutes

Ingredients

- ¾ cup unsweetened almond milk
- ½ tsp vanilla extract
- 1 ½ tbsp ground flaxseed
- 3 tbsp ground almonds
- 6 tbsp unsweetened shredded coconut
- Pinch of sea salt

Directions

1. Add almond milk in microwave safe bowl and microwave for 2 minutes.
2. Add remaining ingredients and stir well and cook for 1 minute.
3. Top with fresh berries and serve.

Nutritional Value (Amount per Serving)

Protein: 4.2 g
Carbs: 8.3 g
Fat: 17.4 g
Sugar: 0.6 g
Calories: 197
Cholesterol: 0 mg

LUNCH RECIPE

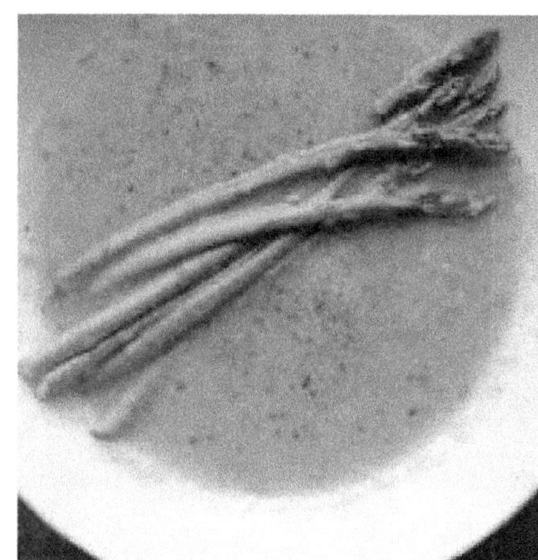

Cauliflower Asparagus Soup

Serves: 4
Prep Time: 30 minutes

Ingredients

- 20 asparagus spears, chopped
- 4 cups vegetable stock
- ½ cauliflower head, chopped
- 2 garlic cloves, chopped
- 1 tbsp coconut oil
- Pepper
- Salt

Directions

1. Heat coconut oil.
2. Add garlic and sauté until softened.
3. Add cauliflower, vegetable stock, pepper, and salt. Stir well and bring to boil.
4. Simmer for 20 minutes.
5. Add chopped asparagus and cook until softened.
6. Stir well and serve warm.

Nutritional Value (Amount per Serving)

Protein: 3.4 g
Carbs: 8.9 g
Fat: 5.6 g
Sugar: 5.1 g
Calories: 74
Cholesterol: 2 mg

DINNER RECIPE

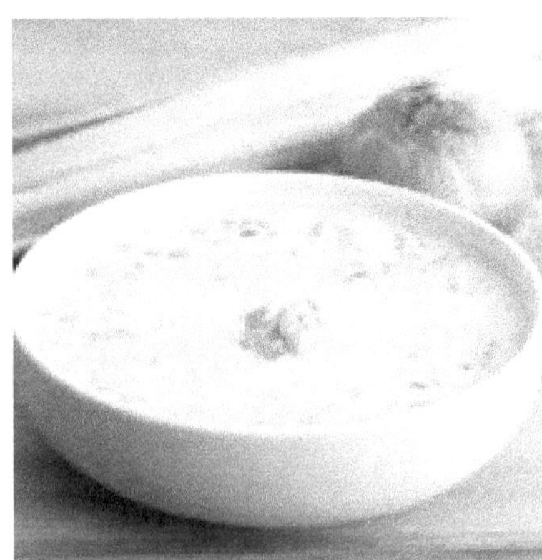

CREAMY CELERY SOUP

Serves: 4
Prep Time: 40 minutes

Ingredients

- 6 cups celery
- ½ tsp dill
- 2 cups water
- 1 cup coconut milk
- 1 onion, chopped
- Pinch of salt

Directions

1. Add all ingredients and stir well.
2. Cover instant pot with lid and select soup setting.
3. Stir well and serve warm.

Nutritional Value (Amount per Serving)

Protein: 2.8 g
Carbs: 10.5 g
Fat: 14.6 g
Sugar: 5.2 g
Calories: 174
Cholesterol: 0 mg

Day 26

Shopping list

- Tofu
- Non-dairy milk
- Onion
- Jalapeno
- Tomatoes
- Cilantro
- Potato
- Tortilla wraps
- Chili powder
- Salt and pepper
- Lemon juice
- Lime juice
- Clove garlic
- Avocado
- Black beans
- Cumin
- Chili powder
- Garlic powder
- Portobello mushroom caps
- Red bell pepper
- Orange bell pepper
- Salt and pepper
- Virgin olive oil
- Spinach
- Potatoes
- Spinach
- Parsley
- Carrots
- Vegetable broth

BREAKFAST RECIPE

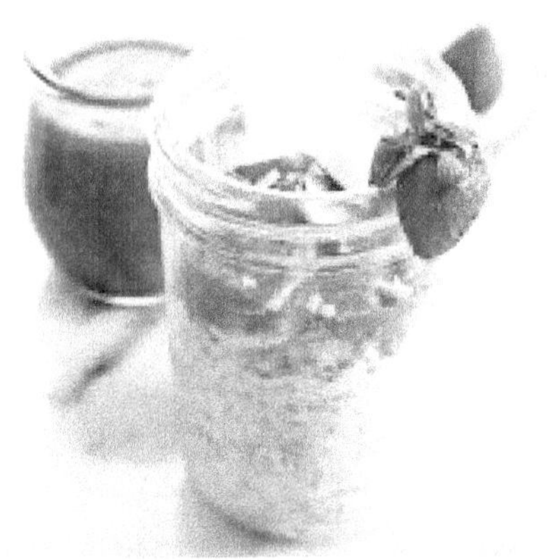

GRAIN-FREE OVERNIGHT OATS

Serves: 1
Prep Time: 10 minutes

Ingredients

- 2/3 cup unsweetened coconut milk
- 2 tsp chia seeds
- 2 tbsp vanilla protein powder
- ½ tbsp coconut flour
- 3 tbsp hemp hearts

Directions

1. Add all ingredients into the glass jar and stir to combine.
2. Close jar with lid and place in refrigerator for overnight.
3. Top with fresh berries and serve.

Nutritional Value (Amount per Serving)

Protein: 27 g
Carbs: 15 g
Fat: 22.5 g
Sugar: 1.5 g
Calories: 378
Cholesterol: 0 mg

LUNCH RECIPE

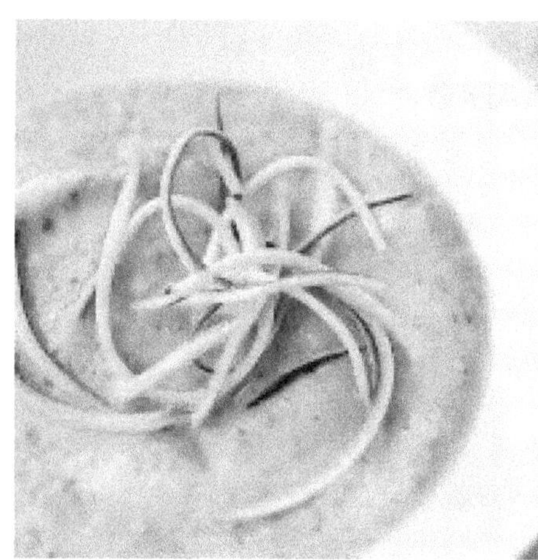

Zucchini Soup

Serves: 8
Prep Time: 20 minutes

Ingredients

- 2 ½ lbs zucchini, peeled and sliced
- 1/3 cup basil leaves
- 4 cups vegetable stock
- 4 garlic cloves, chopped
- 2 tbsp olive oil
- 1 medium onion, diced
- Pepper
- Salt

Directions

1. Heat olive oil.
2. Add zucchini and onion and sauté until softened. Add garlic and sauté for a minute.
3. Simmer for 15 minutes.
4. Remove from heat. Stir in basil and puree the soup using a blender until smooth and creamy. Season with pepper and salt.
5. Stir well and serve.

Nutritional Value (Amount per Serving)

Protein: 2 g
Carbs: 6.8 g
Fat: 4 g
Sugar: 3.3 g
Calories: 62
Cholesterol: 0 mg

DINNER RECIPE

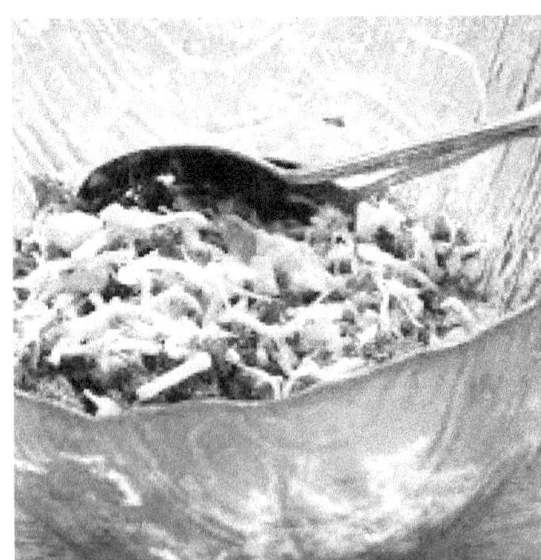

Avocado Almond Cabbage Salad

Serves: 3
Prep Time: 15 minutes

Ingredients

- 3 cups savoy cabbage, shredded
- ½ cup blanched almonds
- 1 avocado, chopped
- ¼ tsp pepper
- ¼ tsp sea salt
- For dressing:

- 1 tsp coconut aminos
- ½ tsp Dijon mustard
- 1 tbsp lemon juice
- 3 tbsp olive oil
- Pepper
- Salt

Directions

1. Mix together all dressing ingredients and set aside.
2. Add all salad ingredients to the large bowl and mix well.
3. Pour dressing over salad and toss well.
4. Serve immediately and enjoy.

Nutritional Value (Amount per Serving)

Protein: 11.6 g
Carbs: 39.8 g
Fat: 14.1 g
Sugar: 9.3 g
Calories: 317
Cholesterol: 0 mg

Day 27

Shopping list

- Tofu
- Non-dairy milk
- Onion
- Jalapeno
- Tomatoes
- Cilantro
- Potato
- Tortilla wraps
- Chili powder
- Salt and pepper
- Lemon juice
- Lime juice
- Clove garlic
- Avocado
- Black beans
- Cumin
- Chili powder
- Garlic powder
- Portobello mushroom caps
- Red bell pepper
- Orange bell pepper
- Salt and pepper
- Virgin olive oil
- Spinach
- Potatoes
- Spinach
- Parsley
- Carrots
- Vegetable broth

BREAKFAST RECIPE

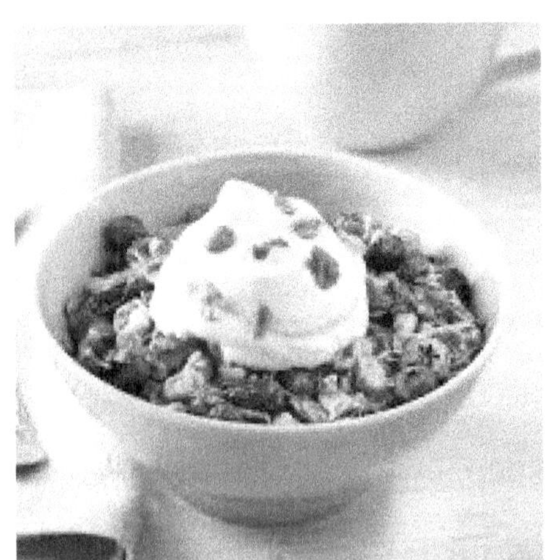

BREAKFAST GRANOLA

Serves: 15
Prep Time: 30 minutes

Ingredients

- 1 tsp ground ginger
- 1 tsp ground cinnamon
- ¼ cups coconut oil, melted
- 1 cup walnuts, chopped
- 2/3 cup pumpkin seeds
- 2/3 cup sunflower seeds
- ½ cup flaxseeds
- 3 cups desiccated coconut

Directions

1. Add all ingredients
2. Spread granola mixture on a baking tray and bake at 350 F/ 180 C for 20 minutes. Turn granola mixture with a spoon after every 3 minutes.
3. Allow to cool completely and serve.

Nutritional Value (Amount per Serving)

Protein: 4.1 g
Carbs: 11.4 g
Fat: 17 g
Sugar: 5.8 g
Calories: 208
Cholesterol: 0 mg

LUNCH RECIPE

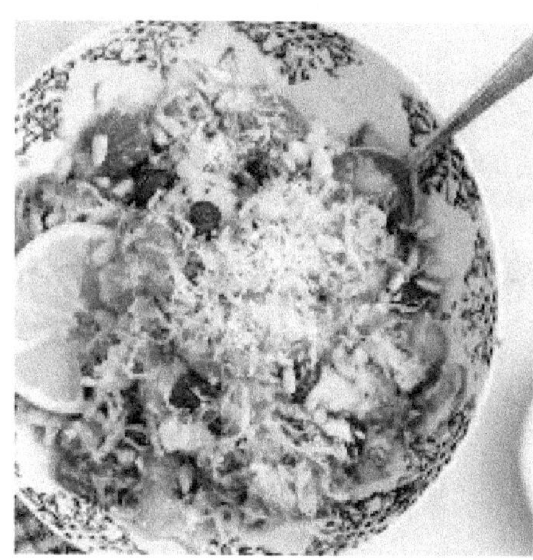

BRUSSELS SPROUTS SALAD

Serves: 6
Prep Time: 20 minutes

Ingredients

- 1 ½ lbs Brussels sprouts, trimmed
- ¼ cup toasted hazelnuts, chopped
- 2 tsp Dijon mustard
- 1 ½ tbsp lemon juice
- 2 tbsp olive oil
- Pepper
- Salt

Directions

1. Whisk together oil, mustard, lemon juice, pepper, and salt.
2. In a large bowl, combine together Brussels sprouts and hazelnuts.
3. Pour dressing over salad and toss well.
4. Serve immediately and enjoy.

Nutritional Value (Amount per Serving)

Protein: 4.4 g
Carbs: 11 g
Fat: 7.1 g
Sugar: 2.7 g
Calories: 111
Cholesterol: 0 mg

DINNER RECIPE

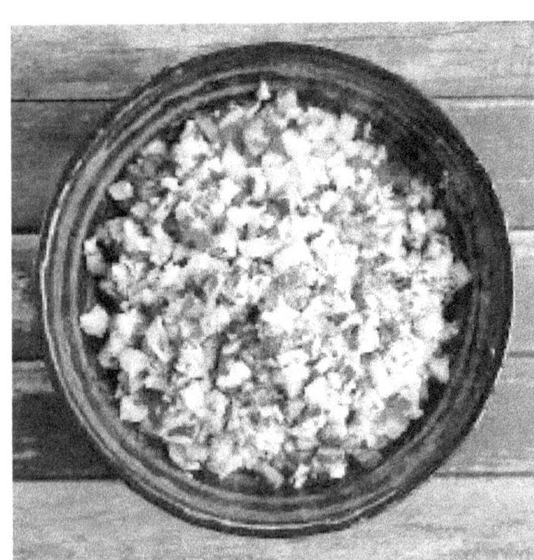

Cauliflower Radish Salad

Serves: 4
Prep Time: 15 minutes

Ingredients

- 12 radishes, trimmed and chopped
- 1 tsp dried dill
- 1 tsp Dijon mustard
- 1 tbsp cider vinegar
- 1 tbsp olive oil
- 1 cup parsley, chopped
- ½ medium cauliflower head, trimmed and chopped
- ½ tsp black pepper
- ¼ tsp sea salt

Directions

1. In a mixing bowl, combine together cauliflower, parsley, and radishes.
2. In a small bowl, whisk together olive oil, dill, mustard, vinegar, pepper, and salt.
3. Pour dressing over salad and toss well.
4. Serve immediately and enjoy.

Nutritional Value (Amount per Serving)

Protein: 2.1 g
Carbs: 5.6 g
Fat: 3.8 g
Sugar: 2.1 g
Calories: 58
Cholesterol: 0 mg

Day 28

Shopping list

- Tofu
- Non-dairy milk
- Onion
- Jalapeno
- Tomatoes
- Cilantro
- Potato
- Tortilla wraps
- Chili powder
- Salt and pepper
- Lemon juice
- Lime juice
- Clove garlic
- Avocado
- Black beans
- Cumin
- Chili powder
- Garlic powder
- Portobello mushroom caps
- Red bell pepper
- Orange bell pepper
- Salt and pepper
- Virgin olive oil
- Spinach
- Potatoes
- Spinach
- Parsley
- Carrots
- Vegetable broth

BREAKFAST RECIPE

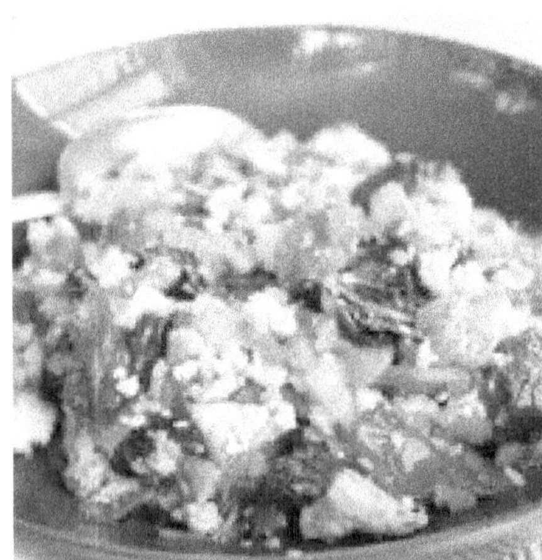

VEGETABLE TOFU SCRAMBLE

Serves: 2
Prep Time: 20 minutes

Ingredients

- 1 block firm tofu, drained and crumbled
- ½ tsp turmeric
- ¼ tsp garlic powder
- 1 cup spinach
- 1 red pepper, chopped
- 10 oz mushrooms, chopped
- ½ onion, chopped
- 1 tbsp olive oil
- Pepper
- Salt

Directions

1. Heat olive oil.
2. Add onion, pepper, and mushrooms and sauté until cooked.
3. Add crumbled tofu, spices, and spinach. Stir well and cook for 3-5 minutes.
4. Serve and enjoy.

Nutritional Value (Amount per Serving)

Protein: 9.6 g
Carbs: 13.7 g
Fat: 9.6 g
Sugar: 7 g
Calories: 159
Cholesterol: 0 mg

LUNCH RECIPE

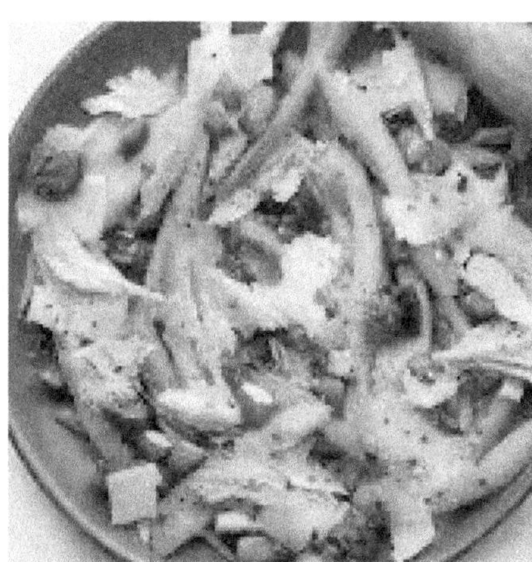

CELERY SALAD

Serves: 6
Prep Time: 10 minutes

Ingredients

- 6 cups celery, sliced
- ¼ tsp celery seed
- 1 tbsp lemon juice
- 2 tsp lemon zest, grated
- 1 tbsp parsley, chopped
- 1 tbsp olive oil
- Sea salt

Directions

1. Add all ingredients
2. Serve immediately and enjoy.

Nutritional Value (Amount per Serving)

Protein: 0.8 g
Carbs: 3.3 g
Fat: 2.5 g
Sugar: 1.5 g
Calories: 38
Cholesterol: 0 mg

DINNER RECIPE

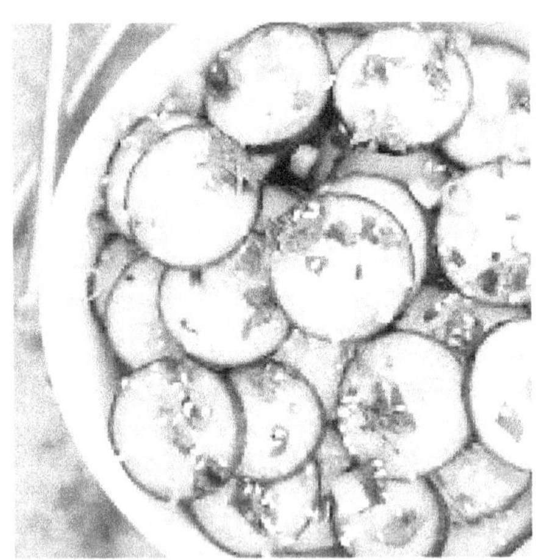

Asian Cucumber Salad

Serves: 6
Prep Time: 10 minutes

Ingredients

- 4 cups cucumbers, sliced
- ¼ tsp red pepper flakes
- ½ tsp sesame oil
- 1 tsp sesame seeds
- ¼ cup rice wine vinegar
- ¼ cup red pepper, diced
- ¼ cup onion, sliced
- ½ tsp sea salt

Directions

1. Add all ingredients and toss well.
2. Serve immediately and enjoy.

Nutritional Value (Amount per Serving)

Protein: 0.7 g
Carbs: 3.5 g
Fat: 0.7 g
Sugar: 1.6 g
Calories: 27
Cholesterol: 0 mg

Day 29

Shopping list

- Tofu
- Non-dairy milk
- Onion
- Jalapeno
- Tomatoes
- Cilantro
- Potato
- Tortilla wraps
- Chili powder
- Salt and pepper
- Lemon juice
- Lime juice
- Clove garlic
- Avocado
- Black beans
- Cumin
- Chili powder
- Garlic powder
- Portobello mushroom caps
- Red bell pepper
- Orange bell pepper
- Salt and pepper
- Virgin olive oil
- Spinach
- Potatoes
- Spinach
- Parsley
- Carrots
- Vegetable broth

BREAKFAST RECIPE

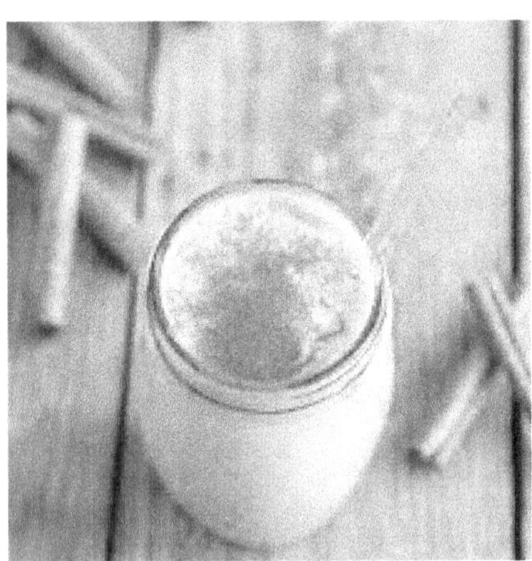

CHIA CINNAMON SMOOTHIE

Serves: 1
Prep Time: 5 minutes

Ingredients

- 2 scoops vanilla protein powder
- 1 tbsp chia seeds
- ½ tsp cinnamon
- 1 tbsp coconut oil
- ½ cup water
- ½ cup unsweetened coconut milk

Directions

1. Blend until smooth and creamy.
2. Serve immediately and enjoy.

Nutritional Value (Amount per Serving)

Protein: 31.6 g
Carbs: 13.4 g
Fat: 23.9 g
Sugar: 0 g
Calories: 397
Cholesterol: 0 mg

LUNCH RECIPE

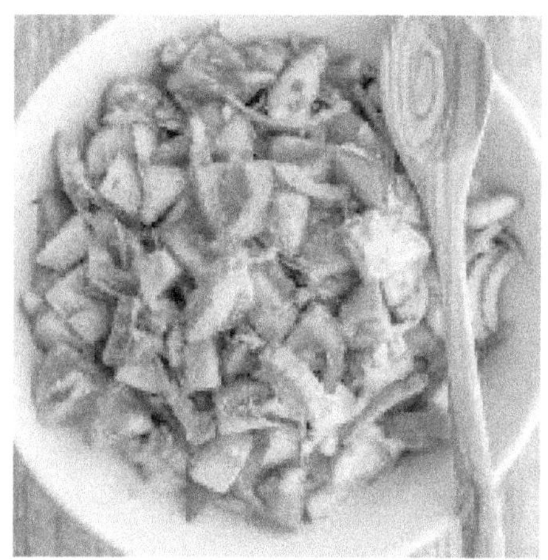

Tomato Avocado Cucumber Salad

Serves: 4
Prep Time: 10 minutes

Ingredients

- 1 cucumber, sliced
- 2 avocados, chopped
- ½ onion, sliced
- 2 tomatoes, chopped
- 1 bell pepper, chopped
- For dressing:

- 2 tbsp cilantro
- ¼ tsp garlic powder
- 2 tbsp olive oil
- 1 tbsp lemon juice
- ½ tsp black pepper
- ½ tsp salt

Directions

1. Mix together all dressing ingredients and set aside.
2. Add all salad ingredients into the large mixing bowl and mix well.
3. Pour dressing over salad and toss well.
4. Serve immediately and enjoy.

Nutritional Value (Amount per Serving)

Protein: 2.1 g
Carbs: 10.6 g
Fat: 9.8 g
Sugar: 5.1 g
Calories: 130
Cholesterol: 0 mg

DINNER RECIPE

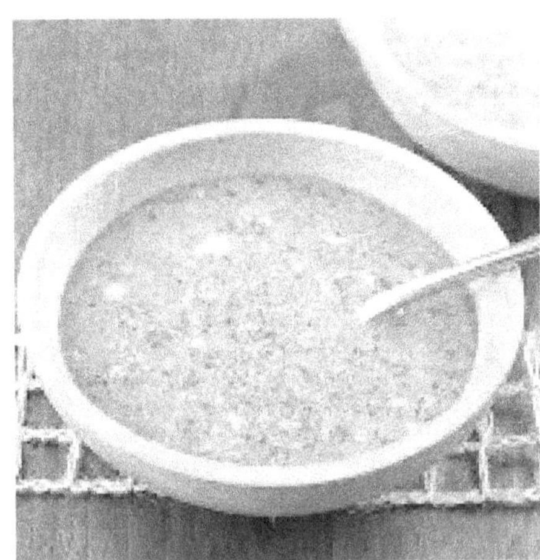

Avocado Broccoli Soup

Serves: 4
Prep Time: 25 minutes

Ingredients

- 2 cups broccoli florets, chopped
- 5 cups vegetable broth
- 2 avocados, chopped
- Pepper
- Salt

Directions

1. Cook broccoli. Drain well.

2. Add broccoli, vegetable broth, avocados, pepper, and salt to the blender and blend until smooth.

3. Stir well and serve warm.

Nutritional Value (Amount per Serving)

Protein: 9.2 g
Carbs: 12.8 g
Fat: 21.5 g
Sugar: 2.1 g
Calories: 269
Cholesterol: 0 mg

Day 30

Shopping list

- Tofu
- Non-dairy milk
- Onion
- Jalapeno
- Tomatoes
- Cilantro
- Potato
- Tortilla wraps
- Chili powder
- Salt and pepper
- Lemon juice
- Lime juice
- Clove garlic
- Avocado
- Black beans
- Cumin
- Chili powder
- Garlic powder
- Portobello mushroom caps
- Red bell pepper
- Orange bell pepper
- Salt and pepper
- Virgin olive oil
- Spinach
- Potatoes
- Spinach
- Parsley
- Carrots
- Vegetable broth

BREAKFAST RECIPE

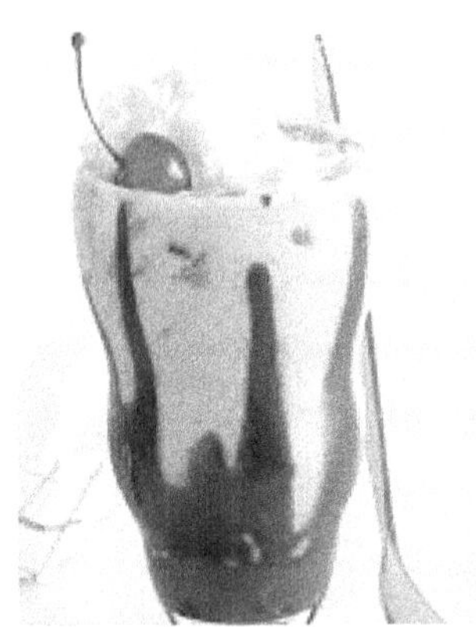

CHOCOLATE STRAWBERRY MILKSHAKE

Serves: 2
Prep Time: 5 minutes

Ingredients

- 1 cup ice cubes
- ¼ cup unsweetened cocoa powder
- 2 scoops vegan protein powder
- 1 cup strawberries
- 2 cups unsweetened coconut milk

Directions

1. Add all ingredients and blend until smooth and creamy.

2. Serve immediately and enjoy.

Nutritional Value (Amount per Serving)

Protein: 27.7 g
Carbs: 15 g
Fat: 5.7 g
Sugar: 6.8 g
Calories: 221
Cholesterol: 0 mg

LUNCH RECIPE

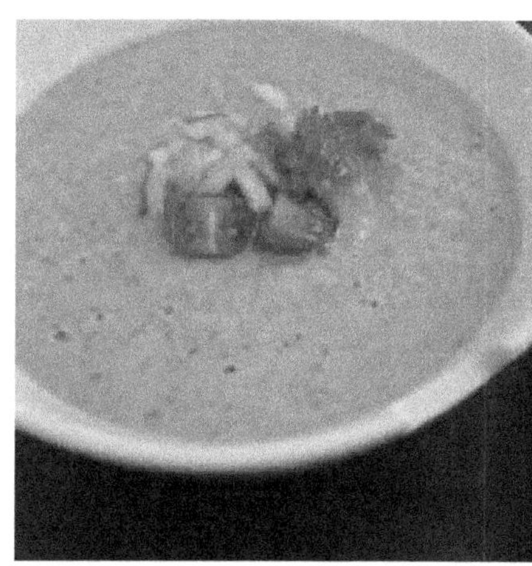

Avocado Cucumber Soup

Serves: 3
Prep Time: 40 minutes

Ingredients

- 1 large cucumber, peeled and sliced
- ¾ cup water
- ¼ cup lemon juice
- 2 garlic cloves
- 6 green onion
- 2 avocados, pitted
- ½ tsp black pepper
- ½ tsp pink salt

Directions

1. Add all ingredients into the blender and blend until smooth and creamy.
2. Place in refrigerator for 30 minutes.
3. Stir well and serve chilled.

Nutritional Value (Amount per Serving)

Protein: 2.2 g
Carbs: 9.2 g
Fat: 3.7 g
Sugar: 2.8 g
Calories: 73
Cholesterol: 0 mg

DINNER RECIPE

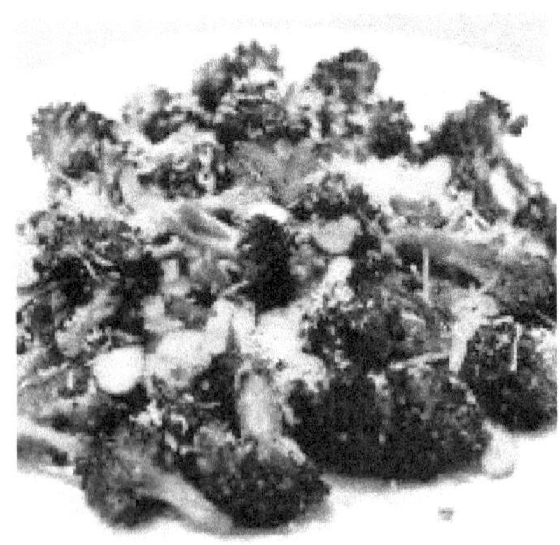

ROASTED ALMOND BROCCOLI

Serves: 4
Prep Time: 25 minutes

Ingredients

- 1 1/2 lbs broccoli florets
- 3 tbsp olive oil
- 1 tbsp fresh lemon juice
- 3 tbsp slivered almonds, toasted
- 2 garlic cloves, sliced
- 1/4 tsp pepper
- 1/4 tsp salt

Directions

1. The oven to be preheated to 425 F/ 218 C.
2. Spray baking dish with cooking spray.
3. Add broccoli, pepper, salt, garlic, and oil in large bowl and toss well.
4. Spread broccoli on the prepared baking dish and roast in preheated oven for 20 minutes.
5. Add lemon juice and almonds over broccoli and toss well.
6. Serve and enjoy.

Nutritional Value (Amount per Serving)

Protein: 5.8 g
Carbs: 12.9 g
Fat: 13.3 g
Sugar: 3.2 g
Calories: 177
Cholesterol: 0 mg

Chapter 6:

Maintaining a progress journal

One thing that I have heard so many people worry and stress about when beginning to adopt a vegan diet is that they will miss the meat, or they're worried about how to get the protein and iron. I've even had so many friends think they couldn't do it because they would miss meat so much and they were scared they wouldn't be able to keep it up over time. So whether you're just becoming a vegan now or you already are one, we're going to tell you how to start on this diet and how to stay on this diet. The one thing I recommend the most is if you're really worried about cutting meat from your diet, go slow. You can be at a dinner with a few friends and they want to share an appetizer and you think one won't hurt, or they want to drink so you figure one drink won't have too many carbs or something along those lines. A quick tip though; a lot of drinks do have carbs and on a ketogenic diet, it is really not recommended because you'll bust straight through your numbers. Some people even give in to the peer pressure because their friends get upset that someone is not eating like the rest of them. Also, if it helps, there are so many yummy alternatives to meat and you can find them at just about any supermarket which should make the switch even easier. Another thing to remind people is that once you begin adjusting to this diet, you will probably begin to crave meat less and less. Many people have said that they have been vegan for most of their lives and don't miss meat at all. Others say they feel bad for the meat eaters who are missing out on what vegetarians and vegans enjoy every day, from the great health benefits of the food to the wonderful flavors of the new foods in their diet.

A good tip to start out is do not go cold turkey. No pun intended. When you go cold turkey without adequate preparation, you tend to be more likely to go back to eating meat and your old diet. Then you feel guilty and it can be a bad cycle. Removing it slowly over time is the best way to go about this because you're familiarizing your body to the new food and letting go of the old. Over time, you'll notice that you're craving meat less and the switch will become easier. A good example to go with is let's say you're trying to cut sweets out of your diet. So you remove anything with sugar in your house. Then you start to eat healthy for maybe a few hours or a day and you begin to get cravings. The problem with many people is that they get so hungry because they don't have the proper research about what to eat, and then they end up going on a binge or running out to the nearest place with cookies or they stay home, and binge eat. Now, you might think binging on healthy food is better but it's not. Binge eating is never healthy and can lead to eating disorders which are a bad thing.

Later, you feel guilty and ashamed which only hurts you and your progress as well as your emotional being. If you slip up, remember you are human. It can happen to anyone and there is no reason to feel guilty or ashamed. Slip-ups happen. It is also important to note that slip-ups will probably happen in the first couple of days and if they do, it's alright. The important thing is that you're trying to better yourself and that you want to change. This is a good thing. Reminding yourself of that will help guide you because you will be able to understand that the effort you're putting forth is something to be proud of and one day you won't slip up at all.

You should also begin adding to your diet before taking things away. Familiarize yourself with how you prepare your new food, how it's stored, and the uses they have. With studying, you will see that many of your items can be used as multipurpose items. Olive oil is great for your skin and hair just as one example of how it can be used in a different way. You should start adding more vegan staples but keep in mind that you're both a vegan and ketogenic, not just one or the other. This means that there are certain things that ketogenic eat that vegans don't; like fish or meat for ketogenic; for vegans, most eat beans or potatoes and starchy foods but ketogenic usually avoid them because of the high carb content. So when adding things to your diet, keep in mind what you need to avoid and what will bring the most benefits to your new lifestyle.

Make sure you stay informed. You need to make sure you've got good information going into this because that will help you know what you can and can't eat, or wear or use on your body. Also, stay up to date on science and studies. People are still researching these diets and lifestyles to give people the correct information. If you stay up to date, you'll be able to see the new information too.

If you feel like you can't do it, remind yourself why you decided to do this in the first place. Remind yourself of the facts. Watch videos online or read studies. They say its harder to slip when you see the facts presented to you and you're watching the consequences of eating meat.

Offer to make dinner for your friends or ask if you can make some vegan dishes to a dinner or party. More often than not, you will see that they're really interested in what you have to say and that they will love how amazing your food tastes. They may even opt to go vegan themselves! A perfect example is let's say all your meat-eater friends are having a dinner party and want you to bring a dessert. Okay, easy peasy. Make them some vegan keto zucchini brownies, or some vegan keto cupcakes and watch them fall in love. I bet you won't even be able to tell that there are healthy vegetables in there and your friends will fall in love.

Make your lifestyle the new norm. Everyone thinks that meat-eating is the norm; switch what it means. Now, this doesn't mean getting in people's faces and being rude or abrupt. Be kind and polite. Be happy in the knowledge that you're making a difference and try to feel compassionate to people no matter what choices they make. If you are content with who you are, it is more likely that people will be open to talking to you about this. They could even begin questioning their own choices. But by simply being an awesome and secure person who's happy in their choices, you'll probably begin to see that your friends want to come to you because they see you so happy and want to know what your secret is.

Finding new items and recipes can be a fun and exciting adventure and a great way to keep yourself on track. We can always learn new things and for a lot of people, going on little adventures can be a lot of fun. Get out and about and see what vegan things you can find around you.

Find inspiration. There are so many celebrities that have taken up the cause and so many other people as well. Doctors, lawyers, teachers; there are so many people now that have joined the vegan move. There are also many organizations that have taken up the movement as well. Be careful with these organizations though and make sure they are on the up and up. Studies have shown that some organizations kill more animals than they save. Or some don't follow the ideas you have for yourself. You need to make sure that you find inspiration that is going to help you. Thanks to social media, you can even be connected to hundreds of thousands of people that have the same lifestyle and desires to help animals as you do. You can ask questions and learn everything you can about the vegan lifestyle. As with anything on social media though, you need to be careful as there are dangers beyond bad advice as some people simply can't be trusted so you'll need to be careful that you don't get hurt.

Grow your own food. This one not everyone can do. But if you can, grow your own food. You could grow the food you eat and earn a deeper appreciation for your food and what's going in your body.

You'll be able to see the work and effort it takes to provide yourself sustenance and you might even help other people try new things because the tastes are different. You can grow anything from vegetables to spices. The really cool thing though is if there's something you want to eat but can't find it anywhere, you can grow it yourself. Now, obviously, if you have to grow it, you won't get it when you want it because it would take weeks or months before it would be ready to eat. However, you will be able to have access to it which is a pretty cool thing to think about. If your garden got big enough, you could share with your finds and family and maybe they would be interested in eating healthier foods for themselves and their family because of your example.

Another surprising thing in this digital age is that you can have groceries delivered to you, even fresh ones in certain cases. This might help people who don't have vegan options near them. It will be easier for you to have it delivered especially if you live far away from the city or you're far from a place that actually carries what you need. Online shopping can also be a great way to try some new snacks as long as you're making sure it's not junk food or overly processed stuff that is going to make you gain a lot of weight. Look for options you know are good.

Remember, this is a journey. If you slip up, forgive and motivate yourself to do better so it won't happen again. If you're tired of the current options you're eating, find/keep trying new recipes and foods that you love. Keep looking around and exploring so that your knowledge keeps expanding. This can be a really fun way to make yourself happy and healthy and make sure that you accomplish the goals that you want to reach for yourself.

Conclusion

Plant-based diet is not as complicated as you think it is and most of the ingredients are easy to get, in fact, you might even plant them at your backyard! Unlike the regular diet ingredients, in a situation where you have to find a specific animal parts, some places may run out of them and you might crave for the dish for God knows how long until the parts are available again. Meanwhile, plant-based ingredients are abundant and could be find at your nearest stores or street vendors, at a much lower cost too!

Making a decision to structure how your plant-based diet is going to look is the first step, and it is going to help you transition from your current diet outlook. This is something that is really personal and varies from one person to the other. While some people decide that they will not tolerate any animal products at all, some make do with tiny bits of dairy or meat occasionally. It is really up to you to decide what and how you want your plant-based diet to look like. The most important thing is that whole plant-based foods have to make a great majority of your diet.

I may not be able to ask people to start eating plant-based foods, but it's good enough to make them aware of the nutrition that they consumed daily in their food plan. Furthermore, I cannot change their mind about how easy it is to cook plant-based meals, but at least they could try these recipes at home and that would make them start pondering on the coolness of practicing a plant-based diet one day.

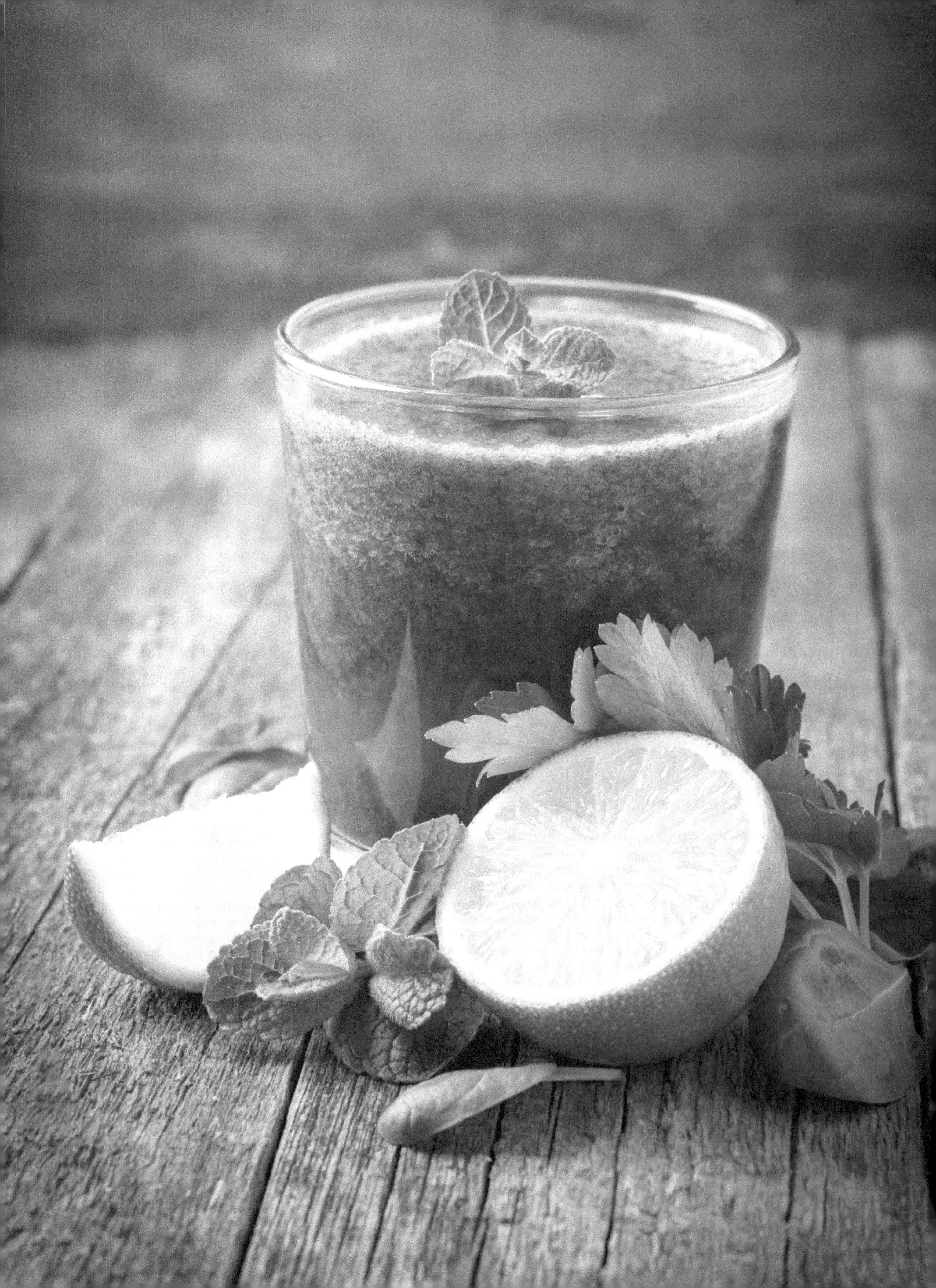